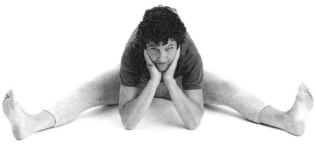

Starting
YOGA

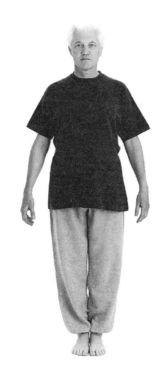

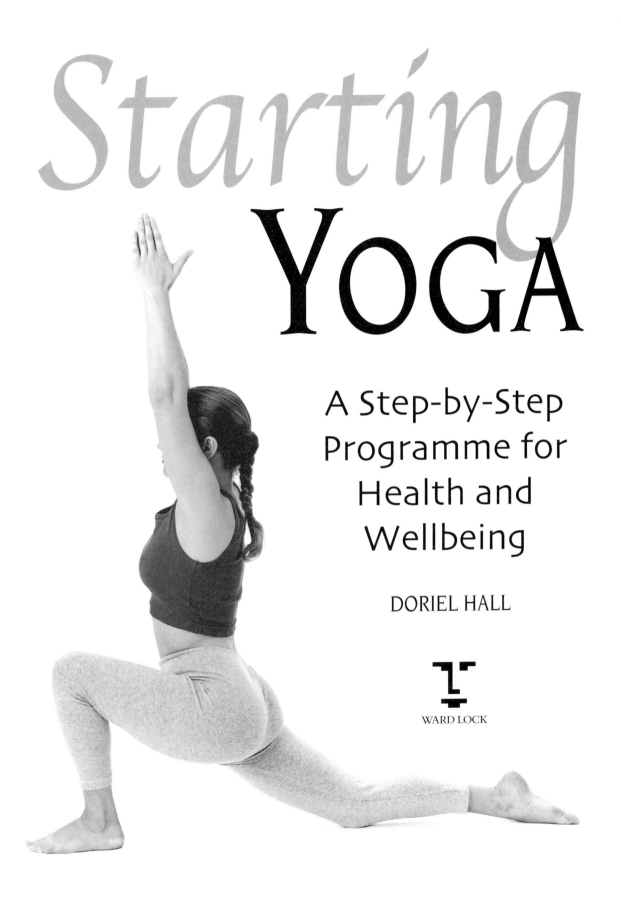

Starting YOGA

A Step-by-Step Programme for Health and Wellbeing

DORIEL HALL

WARD LOCK

To my guru, Paramahansa Satyananda

Thanks to all my teachers, and the students on the British Wheel
of Yoga courses who have taught me so much. Special thanks to
the yogis who modelled for the photographs: Pauline Beakhust
and her sons Matthew and Stephen, Jennifer Eyre, Patricia
Heasman and David Talbot.

First published in the UK 1996 by Ward Lock
Wellington House, 125 Strand
LONDON WC2R 0BB

A Cassell Imprint

Distributed in the United States
by Sterling Publishing Co., Inc.
387 Park Avenue South, New York, NY 10016-8810

A British Library Cataloguing in Publication Data block for this book may be obtained from
the British Library

ISBN 0 7063 7457 6 Pbk
ISBN 0 7063 7751 6 Hbk

Designed by Richard Carr
Printed and bound in Great Britain by The Bath Press

CONTENTS

PART THREE

SPECIFIC AREAS

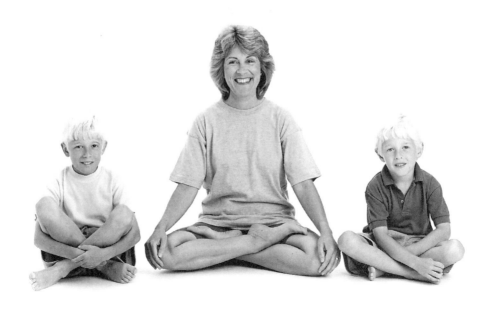

PART ONE

GETTING STARTED

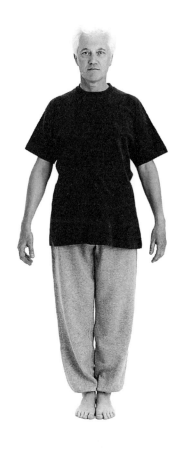

CHAPTER I

WHAT IS YOGA ?

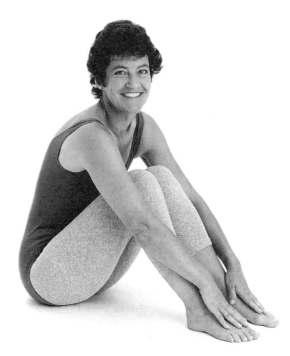

Creating balance and harmony

YOGA TEACHES US to bring all aspects of ourselves and our lives into balance and harmony. Body and mind work together. Different aspects of 'body' – movement and breathing – work together. Different aspects of 'mind' – concentration and relaxation – work together.

We soon begin to notice the difference when we have slipped out of this harmonious way of being. Luckily, wherever we are, no matter what has thrown us off balance, a few discreet yoga breaths or stretches will restore us. People who enjoy yoga recognize each other by their sunny unflappability. It is a good trait to be known by!

THE MEANING OF THE WORD 'YOGA'

The word 'yoga' is Sanskrit – one of the oldest languages in the world which has been called 'the mother of all languages'. It is related to the English word 'yoke'. Yoga yokes the mind to the body, the movement to the breathing, mental focus to relaxation, awareness to activity. This harmonious co-operation brings out the best in us at every level.

'Yoga' is also related to the English word 'conjugal', which describes the 'union between complementary opposites' (as in husband and wife). Mind and body depend upon each other – otherwise no living organism could function at all. Even the most primitive organism has both a structure (body) and an intelligence (mind), however simple and instinctive that intelligence may be. Human minds are both complex and conscious.

Our modern culture is apt to revere the mind at the expense of the body, although they are designed to be equal partners. The result of this imbalance is apparent in all the stress-related physical symptoms that can afflict us. We ignore the human body's needs until our health breaks down. This is a great mistake, for the health of the body influences the health of the mind. Besides, we need bodies for our minds to live in!

'Yoga' is often translated as 'union', as in a marriage. In a good marriage both partners are respected and valued by – and responsive to – each other. In the same way, yoga teaches us to respect the essential unity of body and mind. We become more healthy and whole, as the body responds to the mind's suggestions and the mind is alert and sensitive to the feelings and needs of the body.

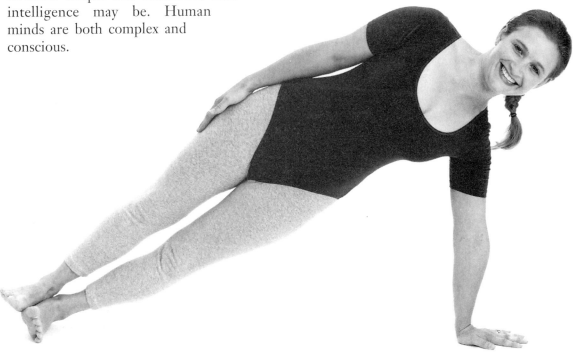

THE AIM OF YOGA

The main purpose of yoga practice is to correct all imbalance and to maintain harmony – between short-term and long-term benefit, between looking outward and looking inward, between exertion and relaxation, between physical and mental activity.

Our modern western lifestyle is very unbalanced in all these areas. We are always in a hurry, forcing ourselves to cope with more and more in less and less time. Inwardness, relaxation and even physical exercise get pushed out of our schedules. We have no time for ourselves.

Even the physical activities that used to be essential for survival are now done by machines, so we take very little physical exercise (compared with our ancestors). Instead, we over-exert our minds. We use them to work the machines that save us time, and spend the time saved on even more mental activity.

Yoga is unique in the way it redresses these imbalances. It makes us focus on how we feel inside ourselves, rather than on what is happening around us. It combines physical activity with mental attention. It teaches us how to live in a state of relaxed exertion rather than in bursts of red alert followed by periods of depressed exhaustion.

BODY–MIND COMMUNICATION

The body and mind communicate with each other via the nervous system or, rather, systems. Our five senses relay to the brain what is going on 'out there' via the sensory nervous system. The brain (the instrument of the mind, or consciousness) then decides how to respond to this information and gives its orders via the motor nervous system. The sensory nerves bring information to the brain through our eyes, ears, nose, tongue and skin. The motor nerves travel from the brain to the body, carrying the brain's instructions.

We may not be conscious of this process – for example, when we scratch an itch or perform complicated sequences of movements that we have learned, such as walking, talking or driving a car. Of course, we also choose to make many movements consciously.

THE AUTONOMIC NERVOUS SYSTEM

Another type of communication system also operates between the brain and the body. This is the autonomic nervous system, which works by releasing chemicals into the bloodstream. It is divided into two branches that have complementary functions, rather like the brakes and accelerator in a car. One branch attends to immediate danger and tries to keep the body safe. The other branch attends to the long-term survival of the body, through nourishment, rest and repair.

We need to maintain a balance between these demands but, since our reactions to ongoing stress have to take precedence, our long-term interests are apt to be set aside in the stressful world we live in. Many vital systems become repressed – immune response, rest and repair – while others become overactive and exhausted.

SAFETY ASPECT OF YOGA

The inner awareness of the body that is developed through yoga practice guards against physical strain and injury, whether practising yoga or any other activity. Yoga gradually develops self-awareness, self-responsibility and self-consideration, whatever we are doing.

This attitude of care and respect for the needs of the body carries over into everyday life. We learn to stand and sit with good posture, to align the joints before lifting heavy objects, and to remain relaxed in mind and body even when we are very active.

Other forms of exercise – such as most keep-fit routines and sports – do not usually include this built-in safety aspect, this self-monitoring, which prevents strain and injury. Any routine that follows brisk music, for instance, or any large class synchronized to the teacher's pace, may not suit some people. Keeping up can be stressful – and dangerous – for anyone who is unused to vigorous exercise, who has a legacy of past injuries, or who feels tired or unwell.

We all need to discover and follow our own inner rhythms. These rhythms are based on our individual breathing patterns, and on our moment-by-moment awareness of our body's response to what is being asked of it. In this way we learn to recognize the signs of strain – and to stop whatever we were doing.

Since yoga is so personal, a good teacher will observe the students carefully and plan each class to suit individual needs. Even so, it is always up to each student to decide how much effort to put in and when to stop and rest. Yoga teaches self-responsibility.

When we are practising without a teacher to guide us, it is especially important to watch out for any signals of strain and to adjust our effort accordingly. Such signals may include laboured or rapid breathing, shaking in the limbs, fatigue, speeded-up heartbeat or feeling hot and bothered – especially in poses where the head is lower than the heart. Detailed reminders of such watchpoints are given throughout this book.

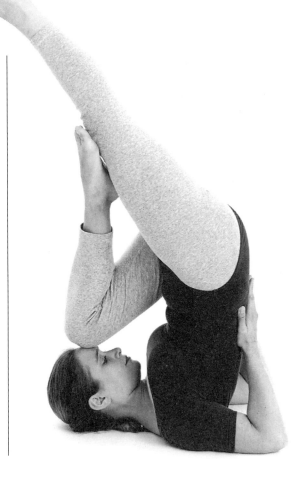

YOGA IS NOT COMPETITIVE

Yoga, unlike most sports, is not competitive. Performance is never judged against anyone else's standards – nor even against one's own achievements on a better or worse day. The only person involved is oneself, the only place is here and the only time is now.

The aim is to maintain a state of relaxed exertion now – and gradually to learn how to extend this 'now' into the whole of one's

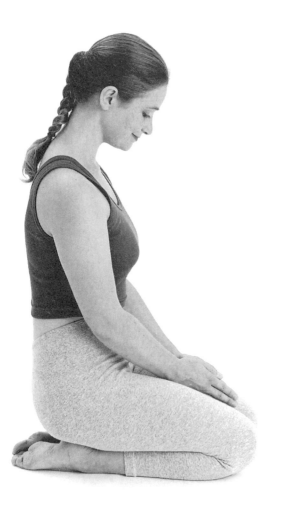

life. Regular practice is needed. A sense of optimism helps, too. Even if we stop practising for a while, for whatever reason, nothing we have done is wasted. It all helps us to build up this one-pointedness, this relaxed focus on whatever it is we are doing.

Eventually, body and mind may be truly united – rather than our bodies doing one thing while our minds are off doing something else! If we can achieve this responsive harmony within our own selves, it is only a small step to achieving it in our relationships to the world and the people around us. Putting the world to rights starts with oneself!

Stress builds up because of this tendency to switch our minds off from the body's natural responses. The body tries to signal ever more loudly, while we feed it pills to silence it and force it to submit to our will! This may lead to physical illness, and also to living almost totally in our heads.

We worry about possible problems in the future, we build castles in the air, we plan and dream. We may even become 'too heavenly to be any earthly use,' while our lives slip by – unlived.

One-pointed focus upon what we are engaged in now, together with a serene and untroubled outlook, actually achieves far more than scurrying around trying to do everything at once!

Many of us have actually forgotten how it feels to relax and to enjoy non-rushed, non-competitive activity. We may have become so used to living with stress – feeling tense, fearful, competitive, even aggressive – that we wonder what is wrong with us if we find ourselves not keyed up and on perpetual red alert! Serenity may take some getting used to.

HOW YOU 'DO' YOGA

Most people new to yoga expect to learn gentle stretching exercises. This is the most 'visible' aspect of yoga practice but there is much more to it than this. The movements are slow and often synchronized with the breathing. The mind is totally focused on how the body is responding. Communication and rapport are being built up between mind and body. All muscles that are not involved are learning to relax. All thoughts that are not relevant fade away gently. A stillness of mind and body is gradually achieved – and from this point we can plunge into the day's activities with renewed vigour. This is why yoga is both energizing and relaxing.

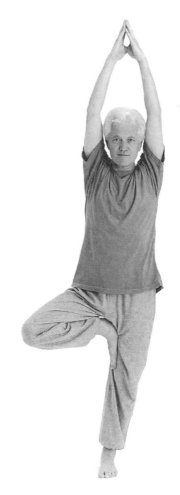

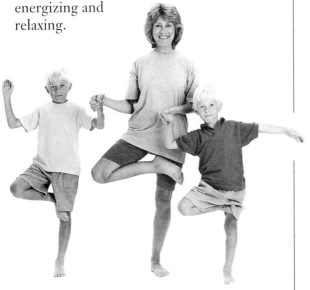

There are many excellent keep-fit routines, often based on yoga exercises. Yoga, however, is designed to be tailored to the individual. Unless body and mind are working together and responsive to each other, yoga is not being practised – however beneficial the exercises may be in themselves.

THE BREATH IS THE KEY

Most of the changes that occur in our bodies, as the result of the activities of the autonomic nervous system, are outside our conscious control. Few people are able to change the rate of their heartbeat or digestion, for instance, or the chemical constituents in their blood.

We can all, however, learn to change our breathing patterns. This directly affects the autonomic nervous system. When we are keyed-up and anxious, our breathing becomes rapid and shallow. Many people always breathe like this. They may have learned this pattern early in life when they were feeling frightened and insecure. Now this breathing pattern keeps them locked into anxiety.

As we learn to breathe slowly and deeply, we are also learning how to relax. In this way we can change our whole outlook on life. Yoga teaches us to become *aware* of our personal breathing patterns, through synchronizing our movements with our breathing. Gradually they both get slower, as the breathing deepens. We learn to focus on the breath, to watch it. This 'inward-looking' makes us feel more relaxed, which deepens the breath even more. Breathing

slowly and deeply is actually the natural way to breathe, helping us to be relaxed and contented with life.

Instructions are given throughout this book on how to synchronize the movements with the breathing. This is the physical aspect of yoga. Linking focus with relaxation is the mental aspect. Joining the physical with the mental aspects is the essence of yoga practice, and the source of all its benefits.

Specific breathing and relaxation techniques are also given, to help us to unwind even more. No wonder so many people swear by yoga, as the antidote to the stresses and imbalances of modern life!

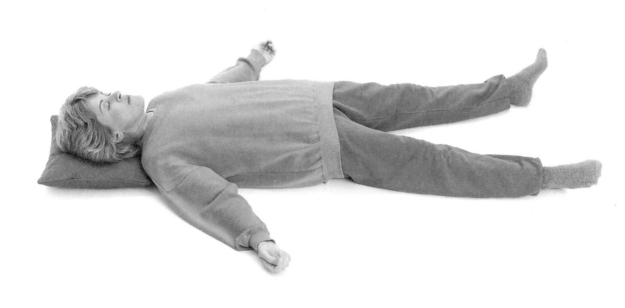

CHAPTER 2

PREPARING TO PRACTISE YOGA

Time, place and clothing

YOGA NEEDS TO be practised regularly, in order for the benefits to build up. It should become as much a part of your life as cleaning your teeth. The best way to get into a regular routine is to set aside the same slot in your day, every day, for yoga practice. Of course life never runs that smoothly! But making yoga a daily habit is the best and easiest way to ensure that you actually practise. Going to a yoga class regularly is also a great help in supporting your private practice. So is the satisfaction you feel as you begin to reap the benefits.

EARLY MORNING YOGA

Since yoga builds up your ability to relax – among its many bonuses – it is best to choose a time when you can expect to be undisturbed. For many people the early morning proves to be the best time. Set your alarm, if necessary, giving yourself enough time to wake up, wash and enjoy a drink before you begin. Before long, yoga practice should be such an agreeable habit that you look forward to this special time to yourself.

Yoga practice first thing in the morning has many advantages. You are relaxed after a good night's sleep. If you practise at the end of a busy day, it may take time and determination to let go of the day's concerns. You will need a longer practice session to achieve the same results.

Also, yoga should be practised on an empty stomach, with empty bladder and bowels. You should wait for two hours after a meal or at least an hour after a light snack. Yoga movements compress the abdomen, so working on a partly digested meal can be most uncomfortable.

The concentration required for yoga practice should not be broken by interruptions. Disconnect the telephone and train the family to respect your special time for yoga. Perhaps you can practise yoga together later on during the day. Children love yoga, but their attention span is short. The yoga you do with them will be great fun but should be an addition to your private practice, not a substitute for it.

OTHER GOOD TIMES TO PRACTISE

If you have small children, mid-morning may be most convenient. If you work at home, yoga before lunch is a wonderful pick-me-up. Some people eat a light snack on the way home from work, and then practise before settling down for the evening. If you are inclined to feel stiff in the mornings, you may prefer to practise later in the day when you have loosened up.

The prime concern is to find a time that suits you, that you can stick to regularly, so that yoga becomes an essential part of your daily life.

THE RIGHT PLACE

Using the same place for practice also helps to develop a routine. Experiment until you find the most suitable spot, then use it every day. Peaceful, positive vibrations will quickly build up there, so that it becomes 'special', a place where you immediately feel relaxed and safe. It can be a small corner, just large enough for your yoga mat or rug. But do make sure that you have room to stretch and move without knocking into anything, so that you can focus within yourself without worrying about your surroundings.

Your mat or rug, kept for yoga, reinforces the feeling that you are entering a special space. It should be non-slip, about 1.8×0.6 m (6×2 ft), so that you can lie down full-length on it. You can buy a special mat for yoga, or use a piece of foam-backed carpet. You will also need a blanket, or extra clothes, to cover you during deep relaxation, as the body temperature drops. A hard foam block or firm cushion is useful when sitting for breathing exercises.

Your 'yoga space' may be enhanced by candles, crystals, flowers or pictures – or it can be

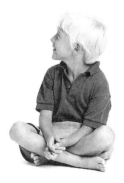

empty and uncluttered. It should be airy, for good breathing, and warm enough for muscles to stretch safely.

CLOTHES

Since yoga is involved with movement of all parts of the body, clothing should be loose and comfortable. Avoid wearing anything made of constricting materials. Cotton leggings or a tracksuit and T-shirt, kept specially for yoga practice, are ideal. Remove jewellery, belts, socks and shoes.

BREATHING

A general principle is to breathe *in* as you stretch the spine *up*. As you breathe *out* you maintain the stretch that you have achieved and either relax or move another part of the body. It may take several slow, deep breaths to get into your best position – for today. The slower the breath-ing, the better – especially the relaxing breath out.

Progress is subtle but surprisingly quick if you practise regularly. You will be astonished how much looser you feel and how much more deeply you are breathing after just a short time. Stretching releases tensions, breathing *in* is energizing and breathing *out* is relaxing.

You may like to imagine a current or stream of light travelling *up* inside you as you breathe *in*, then flowing *down*, right through your whole body, as you breathe *out*. On the way down this stream sweeps away tiredness, tension and stiffness. Working with the breath in this way speeds up progress enormously, for it helps to promote the four aspects of yoga: aware-ness of the body, synchronizing body and breathing, focusing and relaxing the mind. As your breath 'moves' up and down through the body, your mind gets to know your body from the inside – as no-one else can know it. This awareness is your best protection against strain or injury while exercising the body. Yoga is the 'yoking' of body and mind. As you stretch, as you move, as you breathe, always 'keep the mind in the body'.

CHAPTER 3

BASE POSITIONS

Four classical postures

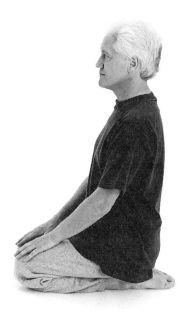

YOGA SEQUENCES OFTEN start from a point of rest, move through various positions to a 'peak', then return to the original position. This makes practice smooth and flowing, like a wave. Each position is an organic development of the previous one – sometimes more demanding, sometimes a variation, sometimes a counter-pose to what has gone before.

The exercises in this book are based on four base positions. The chapter on breathing (page 117–27) introduces another classical posture. The traditional Sanskrit names are used for these positions only; all others are given simple English names. When you go to yoga classes you may find that some teachers use only Sanskrit names. The main thing, however, is to practise, whatever names are used!

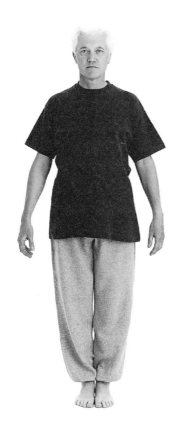

TADASANA

Pronounced *Taad–aah–suhnuh* (*Tada* = mountain, *Asana* = pose). This is the basic standing position, firmly rooted to the earth, like a tree or a mountain. From this 'rootedness' in the feet, the rest of the body stretches upwards in a straight line through the legs, trunk and neck. Good posture creates maximum space in the abdomen and chest, whereas in a slouching position the chest presses on to the abdomen. This restricts both breathing and digestion, and the compression in the spine affects the nervous system. Tiredness and ill-health can result from poor posture.

We stand and walk upright. Only our two feet connect us to the earth. The rest of the body has to stretch upwards from this small support, against the tendency of gravity to pull it downwards. Yoga is always reversing this tendency to slump, by reaching upwards through the spine. Another important principle in yoga is 'joint over joint', so that the weight of the body is distributed evenly and we are poised, ready to move in any direction without creating strain.

To achieve a good Tadasana position, start with your feet, spreading them evenly over the floor to take the weight of your body. They should be parallel, a few centimetres (inches) apart and facing directly forwards. Tight shoes and high heels make us lose our sense of 'groundedness', which is why we practise yoga with bare feet to regain our natural balance. Raising the insteps, if they are slack, aligns the ankles over the heels and cures knock knees – which are due to habitual misalignment – and spreads the weight around the outsides of the feet. This creates a springiness, a lightness of step, that is impossible if the arches are falling inwards.

The next joints to attend to are your knees. They should be directly above your ankles to transfer the weight downwards through the body. They should be loose and poised, not pushed back stiffly, which puts pressure on the lower back. Your hips should be directly over your knees, which may require the pelvis to be tilted and the coccyx (tailbone) tucked under. The pelvis can be thought of as a bowl holding the lower abdominal organs. Often it seems to be tilted, so that everything seems to be spilling out in front. Levelling the rim of the pelvis tucks the tail under, aligns the hips over the knees and reduces a 'sway back' or exaggerated lower spinal curve.

Your navel should be pulled back and up, so that your waist comes directly above your hips, looked at from the side. A long mirror is a help when working on Tadasana, as it is harder to feel misalignment than actually to see it from the side. Next, bring your shoulders in line by raising the sternum (breastbone). The shoulders should be relaxed and dropped, not carrying the whole world. Your arms should hang loosely, not too close to the body or compressing the ribs at the sides. Pull up through the whole trunk, standing tall.

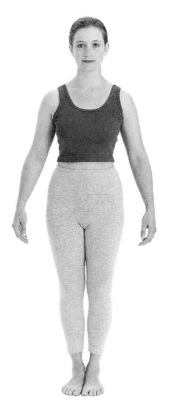

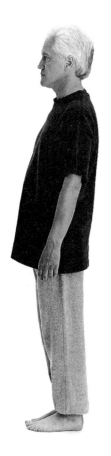

Finally, attend to your head and neck. Tension often tightens the neck muscles at the back, causing the chin to poke forward. Pull your neck back, so that your ears come above your shoulders, seen from the side. Tuck your chin in a little, to lengthen the back of your neck. Look straight ahead – and greet the world with a smile.

The same principles of alignment and 'joint over joint' apply to all yoga practice, so it is well worth spending time improving your Tadasana posture. Say to yourself, 'Tail under, navel up and back, heart lifted and open – and look the world in the eye!' You will be surprised how much better you feel, and how you begin to notice when you are not standing tall. Yoga is meant to influence all of your life, and it does!

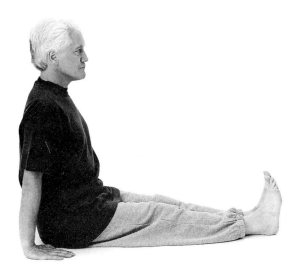

DANDASANA

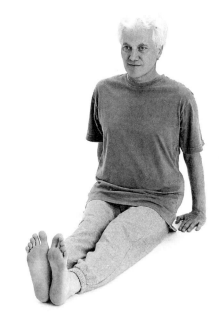

Pronounced *Dand–aah–suhnah* (*Danda* = rod or staff, *Asana* = pose). This is a basic sitting position, with the legs stretched out in front, feet parallel and flexed, toes pointing upwards. Here the legs provide the support, out of which the trunk stretches upwards. Exactly the same principles apply as in Tadasana. The arms are by the sides, shoulders relaxed, with the hands on the floor by the hips, palms down and fingers pointing forward. The trunk is aligned, 'joint over joint', and vertical. The legs are parallel and horizontal.

This pose, like Tadasana, is not as easy as it looks! Most people are stiff in the lower back and hips, so it may take practice – and lots of limbering – to be comfortable with the spine at right angles to the legs and the feet flexed with toes pointing up. The lower back may be contracted through bad posture and tension, or the hamstrings short. A feeling of youth and freedom comes when these tensions are eased!

Concentrate on getting your spine vertical and aligned, as in Tadasana. Feel that you are being pulled up as though by a string attached to the crown.

You may find it helpful, to begin with, to sit on a cushion or foam block. By all means use such help if necessary, but aim to do so on a temporary basis. Practise limbering sequences to loosen the muscles and joints, and check progress before automatically reaching for the cushion. It is so easy to become dependent on external aids, whereas yoga aims at self-reliance through awareness and practice. Keep the rim of the pelvis level, navel pulled back and up, sternum (breastbone) lifted, ears in line with your shoulders, back of your neck long, chin down, gaze level.

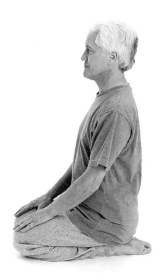

VAJRASANA

Pronounced *Vaj–raah–suhnuh* (*Vajra* = strength (as in the hardness of a diamond), *Asana* = pose). This is the basic kneeling position, or 'sitting on the heels'. Most people find it easier than Dandasana, because the legs are folded rather than stretched out straight. However, there may be pressure on the bones of the feet. If so, put a cushion between your buttocks and heels, or between your feet and the floor. Before long you will not need a cushion, as you loosen up through yoga practice.

To get into Vajrasana, kneel up on the floor. Tuck your coccyx (tail-bone) well under to keep the rim of the pelvis level. Then sit down on your heels, keeping your coccyx

(tailbone) tucked. The heels part naturally, with the buttocks settling between them and big toes touching. Keep your knees together, with your hands on your knees or thighs and palms facing down. This is a very 'contained' position, which is easy to maintain for a long time. Here the folded legs provide the grounding and support, out of which the spine stretches upwards, as in Tadasana and Dandasana.

The stretching of the spine is the most important 'movement' in yoga. It comes first, in the basic starting position from which the other postures follow. It should be maintained, whatever the limbs may be doing. Some postures stretch the front of the spine by bending the trunk backwards. Others stretch the back of the spine through bending forwards. Others rotate the spine, or bend it sideways. However, the spine is always stretched upwards *first*.

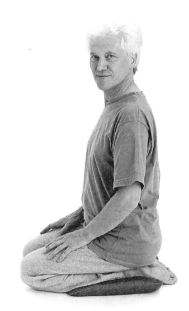

SHAVASANA

Pronounced *Shaa–vaah–suhnuh* (*Shava* = corpse (total stillness of the body), *Asana* = pose). This is the basic lying-down position, from which many sequences start. It is also the best posture for deep relaxation. In this position there is total support, and no reaching upwards. However, there is still alignment and stretching, before encouraging all the muscles to relax. The body remains still and at rest, while the mind remains awake and alert.

rim level, so that your spine is in alignment. You may find that you have to bend your knees slightly but, as your lower back relaxes, your legs will gradually sink to the floor. If you feel strain in your lower back, place a cushion under your legs wherever it is most comfortable. Pull your navel back towards the floor, lift your sternum (breastbone), lengthen the back of your neck and tuck your chin in.

Lift your head and look down along your body to check that you are lying in a straight line. The body's tensions often cause it to lie

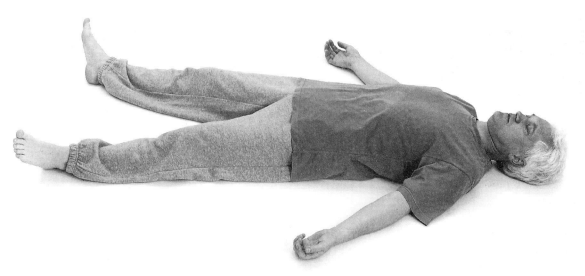

Shavasana involves more than just lying down on the floor on your back!

Place your legs symmetrically apart, with at least 60 cm (2 ft) between your heels. Your toes should roll slightly outwards. This position actually starts in the hip joints. Roll your legs outwards and inwards from your hips, until you find the most comfortable angle for your feet.

As in the previous postures, tuck your coccyx (tailbone) under to bring the pelvic

lopsided. Lower your head, keeping your chin tucked in gently. You may like to use a cushion under the back of your head until your neck releases its tension, if your chin is inclined to poke upwards.

Your arms should lie symmetrically, with your hands about 23 cm (9 in) from the sides of your body and the palms turned up with fingers slightly curled. Rotate your arms at the shoulders until you find the most comfortable position and let your arms rest there. Close your eyes and become aware of the natural breathing process. After a while you may like to take a few focused breaths *up* the body as you breathe *in* and let the breath flow *down* through the body, so that you let go and sink into the floor, as you breathe *out*. If possible, make the breath *out* longer than the breath *in*. With continued practice, deep relaxation can be achieved in the space of three breaths.

Now you are really practising Shavasana! From here you can start on a gentle limbering routine, or a deep relaxation. If you feel tired, weak or unwell, start your yoga practice from Shavasana. You can stretch your body without effort, fully supported by the floor.

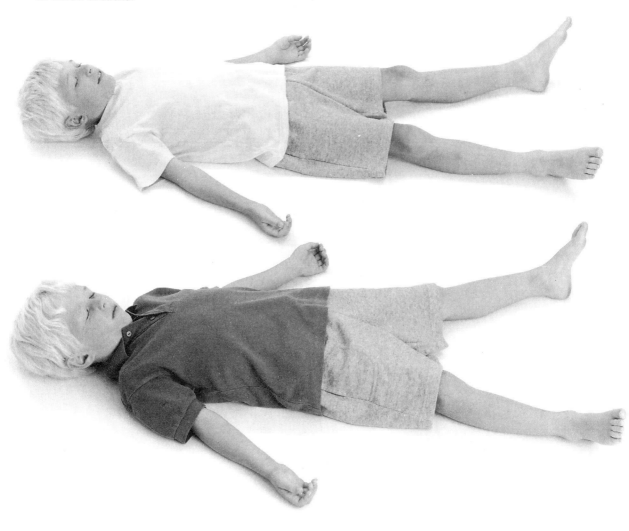

PART TWO

LOOSENING UP

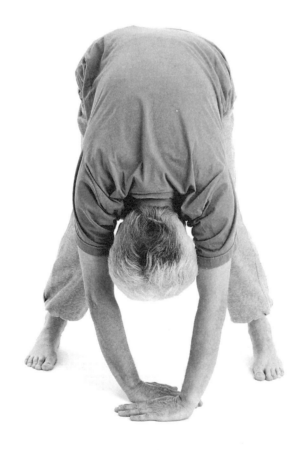

CHAPTER 4

SWITCHING ON THE MIND

Balance and breath

SINCE YOGA IS the 'yoking together' of body and mind, it is good to start with a standing balance. This focuses energy in the head. Yoga always depends on personal experience through practice, so it may take time to develop the sensitivity to 'feel energy'. Meanwhile, there is a simple explanation, for yoga is always practical.

Our balancing mechanisms are situated in the inner ear, within each side of the head. They consist of three canals filled with fluid: one vertical, one horizontal and one transverse. The position of the fluid in these canals tells us which way up we are.

Our eyes also supply information about how we are placed in space. The view is transferred from the eye, via the optic nerve, to the 'seeing' part of the brain at the back of the head. A standing balance, therefore, concentrates a lot of energy in the head,

stimulating what yogis call the 'mind centre' or 'third eye'.

Try shaking your head vigorously, to disturb the inner ear fluids. You will find it hard to balance. It is also difficult to stand on one leg with your eyes shut. A heavy cold or other pressure in the head affects balance, and so does impaired hearing or sight.

A sense of balance, both physical and psychological, gives confidence and clarity to body and mind. We also want to relax, so we focus on our breathing. This brings us directly to the heart of yoga: physical movement and breath 'yoked' to mental focus and relaxation.

Following are three sequences of standing balances. The breathing exercises in Chapter 13 can be an alternative start to yoga practice, as they also sharpen and focus the mind.

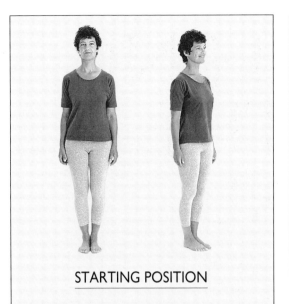

STARTING POSITION

Stand in Tadasana (see Chapter 3 for detailed instructions). Briefly, align your body with the spine erect. Stretch *up* on each breath *in*. Relax your shoulders, arms and face as you breathe *out*. Maintain and improve your position for a few breaths.

ANTELOPE

1 Breathe *out* as you bend your knees and rise on to your toes, keeping the feet parallel. Breathe *in* as you raise your arms to shoulder height and stretch them out parallel in front of you. Hold this position for as many natural breaths as possible. The lower you bend your knees, the higher you raise your heels, and the further you reach forward with your hands, the harder you will work!

WATCHPOINT: Keep the spine vertical in all the stages of the Antelope.

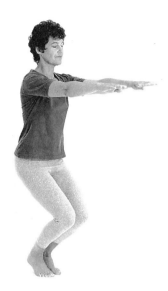

2 Keeping your spine and legs in the same position, bring your hands into the 'Indian greeting' position – palms and fingers together, thumbs joined in front of the sternum (breastbone). Press into the palms with your elbows out to the side. This exercises the arm muscles. Hold this position for several natural breaths. Breathe *out*.

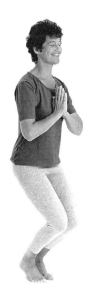

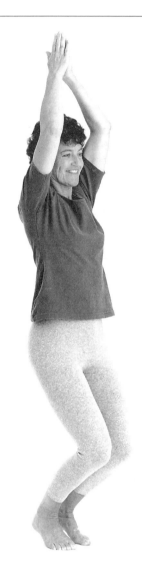

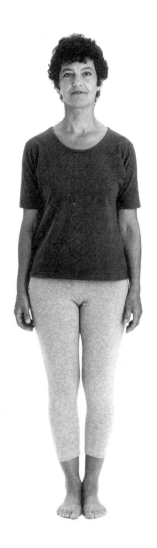

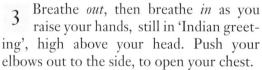

3 Breathe *out*, then breathe *in* as you raise your hands, still in 'Indian greeting', high above your head. Push your elbows out to the side, to open your chest.

Breathe *out* as you return your hands to heart level and in as you take them overhead. Repeat these two movements, until you feel you are about to lose either your balance or your concentration. Before this happens, bring your hands to heart level, straighten your legs and lower your heels.

Stand in Tadasana, and observe yourself from within. What do you feel? Aching limbs? Do they shake? Can you feel a buzz of energy? If so, where? How quickly does your breathing slow down? Can you feel your heart beating? Allow your breathing and your heartbeat to return to a state of rest before you go on to another sequence.

It is important always to ask yourself these questions – and to listen to the answers! In this way you keep within your own safety limits and learn how to extend them. You will be amazed how quickly you can tone up your body and mind with simple movements such as these. The Antelope tones abdominal, leg and buttock muscles. It also works on the chest and arms, and the muscles that uphold the spine. Can you feel this yourself?

RAISED SQUATS

This pose sequence stretches the whole body. It strengthens the legs, lower back and abdominal muscles. It also opens the chest and improves concentration and balance. If you find it difficult to keep the trunk vertical throughout, you can work against a wall. The heels should be about 15 cm (6 in) away from the wall, so that your head, shoulders and buttocks can slide up and down the wall, keeping in contact with it all the time.

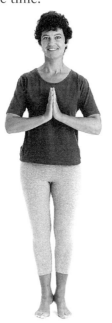

1 Get into a good Tadasana position. Bring your toes out to the sides, about 45 degrees, keeping your heels touching. This is important, so that your knees will bend in alignment with your hips, ankles and toes ('joint over joint') for stability and safe use of the body. Rise on to your toes, keeping heels together. Bring your hands to the 'Indian greeting' position at heart level. Get your balance, with natural breathing.

2 Keeping your spine vertical, bend your knees to the sides and squat on (or close to) your heels as you breathe *out*.

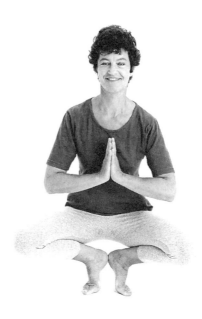

3 As you breathe *in*, stretch up and open your arms to the side, elbows at shoulder level and forefingers touching thumbs. This sweeping movement opens the chest, for better breathing. As you breathe *out*,

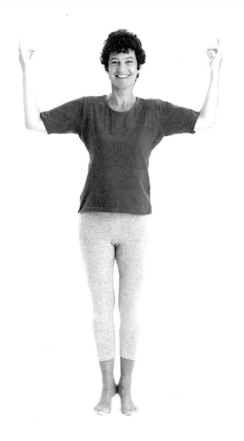

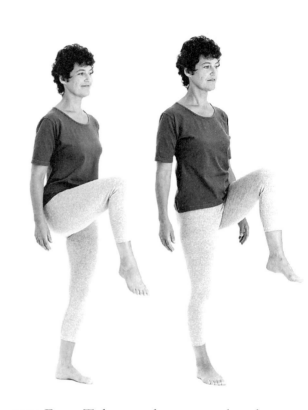

SHAKE A LEG

return to the squatting position. Repeat these two movements, synchronized to your breathing, until you feel you have done enough.

Then return to Tadasana and practise self-observation, as outlined on page 28, until you feel rested.

Both the above sequences are quite energetic and demanding, but at least you are balancing on two feet! In the next sequence you stand tall on one foot only, while swinging the other leg as loosely as possible. The trunk and arms should not move at all. Keep your shoulders, arms and face relaxed throughout. When you have finished the sequence on one side, repeat, standing on the other foot. This is a strong sequence, excellent for getting fit.

1 From Tadasana, choose your best leg to stand on. We all know which one it is! Raise the other knee as high as possible and keep it there. Stretch up through the whole body on the side you are standing on, pulling your waist up out of your hips and your ribs up away from your waist.

With your raised foot dangling loosely from the ankle, swing it back and forth – without moving your raised leg at all, or the rest of your body. The aim is to loosen the ankle joint only.

WATCHPOINT: Stand still and tall throughout the sequence. Natural breathing throughout.

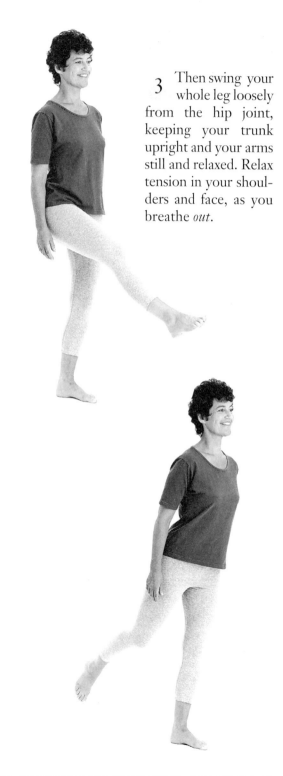

3 Then swing your whole leg loosely from the hip joint, keeping your trunk upright and your arms still and relaxed. Relax tension in your shoulders and face, as you breathe *out*.

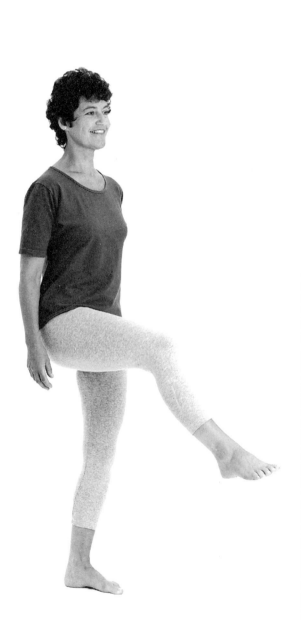

2 Then swing your lower leg loosely back and forth from the knee. Keep the body still and the knee as high as possible. Keep stretching upwards from your standing leg.

Reverse the previous movements, still standing on the same leg. Swing from the knee, then the ankle. Take a deep breath *in*, pulling up the whole body. As you breathe *out*, bring the raised foot to the floor and stand firmly on it. Breathing *in*, raise the other foot and knee and repeat the entire sequence.

When you have finished, return to Tadasana, rest and practise self-observation – keeping your mind in your body – until heartbeat and breathing are completely relaxed. Continue with your yoga practice, feeling balanced, centred, focused and alert.

RAG DOLL

You may like to flop forward, with knees well bent, and swing your trunk and arms loosely from side to side to relax after stretching up in the above exercises.

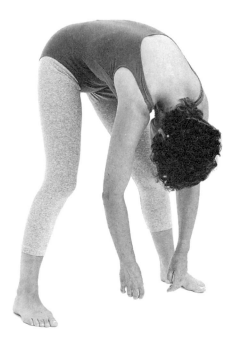

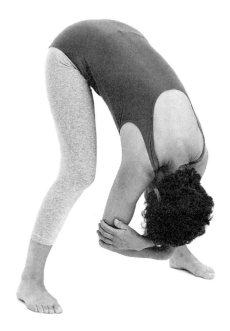

CHAPTER 5

FLOOR STRETCHES

Let gravity support you

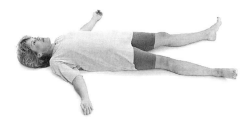

Y OU WILL NOW need to turn your attention to limbering movements. Almost everyone needs to loosen up, to stretch and warm muscles before attempting any very demanding exercise. How much limbering you need, and what type, depends on many factors.

You may feel refreshed and relaxed after a good night's sleep. After your standing balances you may therefore want to limber up from a strong standing position. Or you may be feeling tired, stressed, stiff, out of practice or even unwell. Your body may shudder at the thought of vigorous activity. If so, use the force of gravity to support you as you exercise. Standing exercises are the most taxing, whereas lying-down ones are the most restful.

You will quickly feel more alive, for the following exercises stimulate energy flow in the spine as well as loosening the joints and warming the muscles. They work from the base of the spine upwards, through the sequence as it is given below. Go through them in the order given, even if you only have time to do each movement just a few times. If you feel particularly tight in one area, repeat the relevant exercise a few more times.

By the end of the sequence you will have had a balanced workout, and can safely go on to more demanding exercises if you wish. Even if you have done enough for today, you will still be feeling a great deal better than when you started! Regular practice of this sequence brings amazing results, reducing aches and stiffness and increasing flexibility. It makes you feel younger and fitter and more at home in your body, and the exercises become easier and easier to do.

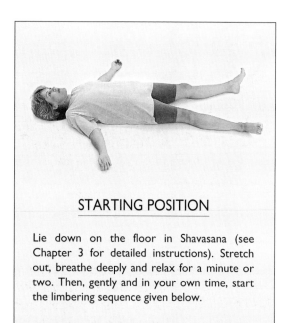

STARTING POSITION

Lie down on the floor in Shavasana (see Chapter 3 for detailed instructions). Stretch out, breathe deeply and relax for a minute or two. Then, gently and in your own time, start the limbering sequence given below.

FOREHEAD TO KNEE

This movement stretches the whole of the spine. It works the hips and upper back and relieves contraction (due to tension) in the lower back and neck, which creates pain and poor posture, adding to the tension. Regular practice reverses this vicious cycle.

1 Bend your right leg, bringing your knee as close as you can to your chest, while keeping your coccyx (tailbone) in contact with the floor. Clasp your hands loosely around the shin of the bent leg, ready to pull down on it.

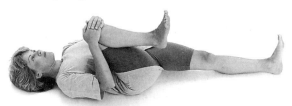

Keep your left leg fully stretched, with the knee straight and the foot flexed, toes to ceiling. In this position breathe *in*.

WATCHPOINT: In any exercise which compresses the abdomen, as this will, it is usual to start on the right side. This is to encourage the natural movement of digestion, which pushes the contents through the large intestine up the right side of the abdomen (from the appendix), across the top and down the left side (to the rectum). Many yoga exercises and positions help to avoid constipation.

2 Breathe *out*, as you lift your head, keeping your chin tucked in and the back of your neck loose and relaxed. At the same time, squeeze your right leg against your chest, so that the knee and forehead meet – or approach each other! Maintain the stretch through your left leg and foot.

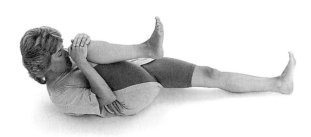

WATCHPOINT: This exercise removes tightness and tension from the shoulders and the back of the neck provided you keep your chin tucked in all the time, so that the back of your neck can stretch. Tension makes it contract, causing the chin to jut out and up.

Breathe *in*, loosen the pull on your right leg and lower your head back to the floor, still keeping your chin tucked in and your left leg stretched. Repeat these movements, synchronized with your breathing, up to six times. Then lower the right leg, stretch out in Shavasana and observe how you feel – especially in the hips, pelvis and neck.

Repeat the same number of times on the other side, with your left leg bent and your left knee over your chest. When you have finished, stretch out again in Shavasana and observe how you feel. Are you balanced on both sides, or does one side need a little more work? If so, repeat a few times on that side, until your body feels balanced.

> WATCHPOINT: None of us are born exactly symmetrical. We may favour one side of the body more than the other. The awareness cultivated by yoga practice helps us to iron out many imbalances that may be causing strain. So it is always important to repeat any one-sided movement equally on the other side and then check whether both sides of the body feel the same.

In the next few exercises you are supported by the arms, shoulders and head. They should relax and not move at all as you twist in the lower part of the body.

FOOT TO SIDE

1 Take your arms out to the side, below shoulder height and well away from the body, palms up. Place your right heel between, or on, the toes of your left foot. Breathe *in*.

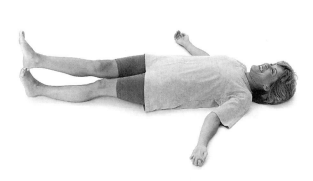

2 As you breathe *out*, bring the joined feet to the floor on the right side. Breathe *in* as you bring them up again, and out as you drop them to the left side (more difficult!). Go as far as you can without strain, letting gravity help you. Breathe *in* as you bring them up again to centre.

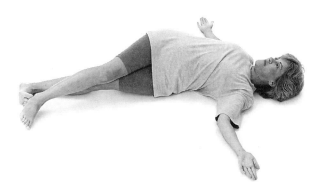

Repeat the sequence a few times, then rest in Shavasana and observe how you feel.

Rest the heel of your left foot on the toes of your right foot and repeat the sequence the same number of times.

KNEE TO SIDE

1 Place your right foot against your left knee, and repeat as in Foot to Side, above. This movement stretches more, slightly higher in the spine. Do only what you can. Flexibility in the hips and spine improves rapidly with regular practice. This whole series should be as relaxed as possible, in order to ease out existing tensions. Do not create more tension by forcing yourself to be flexible!

2 Breathe *out* as you lower the knee to the right side. Breathe *in* as you raise it up again, and out as you lower it as far as possible to the left.

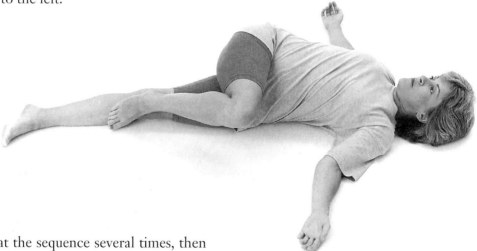

Repeat the sequence several times, then rest in Shavasana and observe how you feel.

Repeat the complete sequence with your left foot against your right knee.

KNEE ROLLS

1 Bend both knees. Plant both your feet as close to your buttocks as possible and wide apart. Breathe *in*. As you breathe *out*, lower both knees to the right, on to the floor.

2 As you breathe *in*, lift both knees to centre and, as you breathe *out*, lower them both to the right, on to the floor. This movement stretches the muscles in the thighs, which are often unconsciously contracted through tension. It makes one feel light and 'springy' in the legs. It may take a bit of practice to reach the floor with both knees.

Repeat several times on each side, until the upper legs feel soft and relaxed.

3 The same movement can be done with knees and feet together, which makes it easier. Do not let them fall apart, but use your inner thigh muscles to keep the legs 'glued' together. The twist in the spine is moving up with each sequence. Can you feel this?

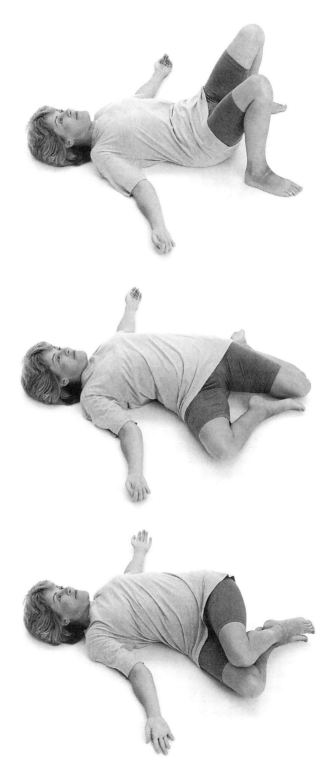

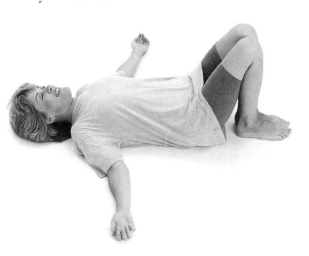

KNEES TO CHEST

1 Raise one knee at a time (especially if your back is weak) and make sure that your whole spine, including your coccyx (tailbone), remains on the floor to support you. When both knees are up, breathe *in*.

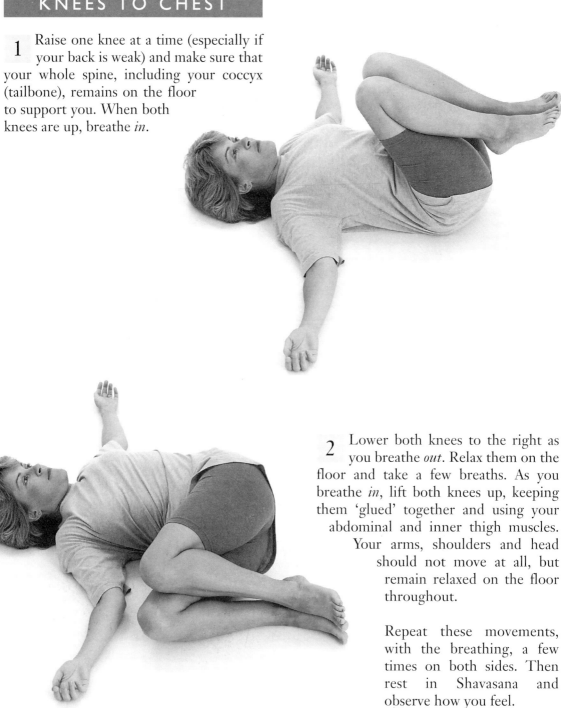

2 Lower both knees to the right as you breathe *out*. Relax them on the floor and take a few breaths. As you breathe *in*, lift both knees up, keeping them 'glued' together and using your abdominal and inner thigh muscles. Your arms, shoulders and head should not move at all, but remain relaxed on the floor throughout.

Repeat these movements, with the breathing, a few times on both sides. Then rest in Shavasana and observe how you feel.

The next version of Knees to Chest opens the chest and relieves tension in the shoulders and upper arms.

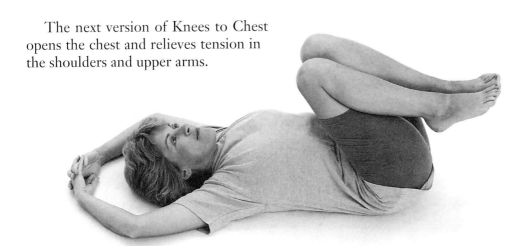

1 With your back flat on the floor and both knees already over your chest, change your arm position. Ideally, the hands should be clasped together several centimetres (inches) behind your head, with your elbows resting on the floor. This may take practice! The head, shoulders and arms provide support and remain unmoving, as before.

2 Move your knees up to centre as you breathe *in* and down to the floor at the side as you breathe *out*, alternating sides, until you feel tired. Then rest in Shavasana and observe how you feel.

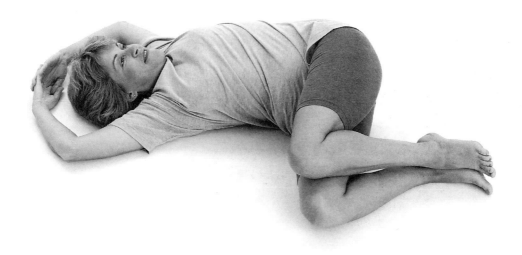

UNIVERSAL POSE

This pose stretches the top half of the body, especially the upper back, shoulders and neck which have been motionless supports up until now. The lower half of the body now becomes the relaxed, unmoving support.

1 From Shavasana roll on to your front, face down. Raise the bent right knee as far up the body as you can, to about waist level, and as far away from you as possible, putting all your weight on to the knees so that you are still lying more on your front than your side. Anchor this knee firmly to the floor with your left hand. Bend your left leg slightly, so that it is comfortable and relaxed. Bring your right hand to join the left. Gaze at your right hand.

2 Breathe *in* as you sweep your right hand and arm around and up, maintaining contact with the floor if you can. Watch your hand, so that your neck, head and eyes also rotate. As you reach the furthest point in this circle, start to breathe *out*, bringing the arm down behind you and back on to your bent knee, gazing at it all the way.

You may find that you cannot keep both the bent knee anchored and the hand in contact with the floor. If this is the case, let your arm rise naturally as it travels round. You will loosen up very quickly with practice, and feel much more open and free around the chest, neck and shoulders as a result.

WATCHPOINT: You do need to keep the bent knee anchored to the floor, or the upper body cannot stretch and the purpose of the movement is lost.

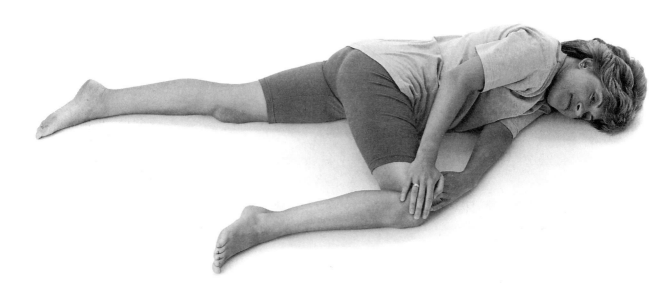

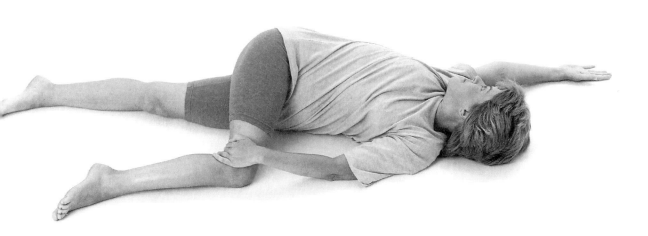

Repeat the movement with your right arm several times, synchronizing it with your breathing. If you are comfortable in the fully extended position, hold that for a few slow breaths, relaxing and releasing through the pectoral muscles in the chest. Then return slowly to Shavasana and observe how you are feeling, before rolling over on to your front again.

Raise the bent left knee up and away from the body and repeat Steps 1 and 2 on the other side.

Rest in Shavasana for a few moments before continuing, or ending, your practice. This resting time between postures is very valuable, provided you keep your mind in your body (see Chapter 13 for deep relaxation techniques).

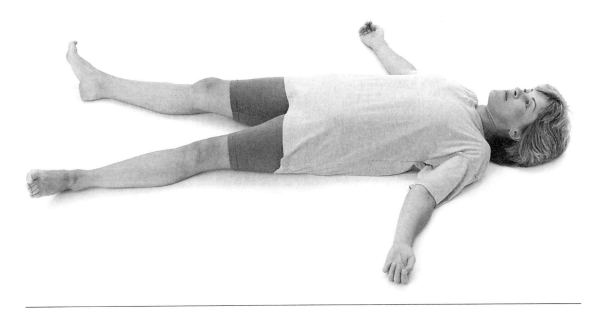

CHAPTER 6

SEATED LIMBERING

Stretching upwards

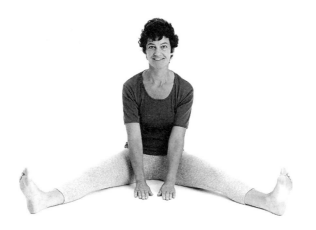

THE STANDING BALANCES in Chapter 4 were stretches with very little support, whereas the sequences in Chapter 5 done lying down had maximum support from the floor. The following seated exercises are well-supported, but also involve plenty of upward stretch.

Weakness, poor posture and an aching lower back are all greatly eased by strengthening the 'lower front'. The spine is held in place by muscles at both the back and the front of it. Lack of exercise, too much sitting and the stretching effect of childbirth can all make the lower abdominal muscles slack, which encourages the lower

back muscles to contract more than they should. Tension also causes tightness in the lower back. The exercises in this chapter quickly re-balance muscle tone in the legs and spine, reversing the damage that may have been building up for years.

WATCHPOINT: Remember to tuck your coccyx (tailbone) under, pull your navel back and lift your sternum (breastbone) up every time you breathe *in*. This makes more space in the abdomen and chest for deeper and fuller breathing, relieves congestion and frees the vertebrae from compression.

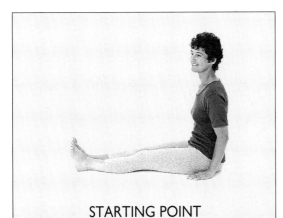

STARTING POINT

Sit down on the floor in Dandasana (see Chapter 3 for detailed instructions). Work to achieve a good position, with spine vertical, legs straight and together, feet flexed and toes pointing to the ceiling. Breathe *in* as you stretch *up*.

JACKKNIFE

This exercise prepares the legs and back for stronger forward bends and creates a feeling of looseness in the hips and lower back.

1 Bring your arms up in front of you at shoulder level, hands a few centimetres (inches) apart with palms facing the floor. Your arms should remain parallel to the floor throughout the sequence and your feet should remain flexed. You need to be aware of the whole body all the time. Your straight legs are the support from which you will stretch upwards, forwards and backwards. Breathe *in* as you stretch *up* through the spine.

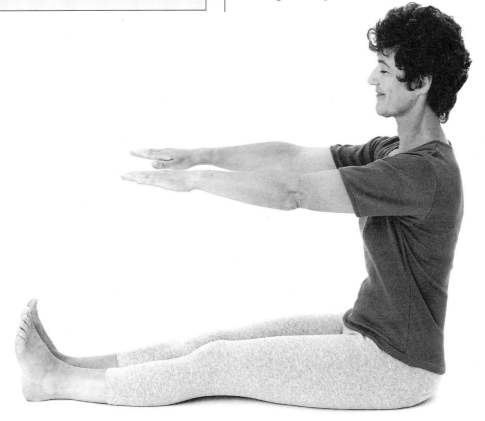

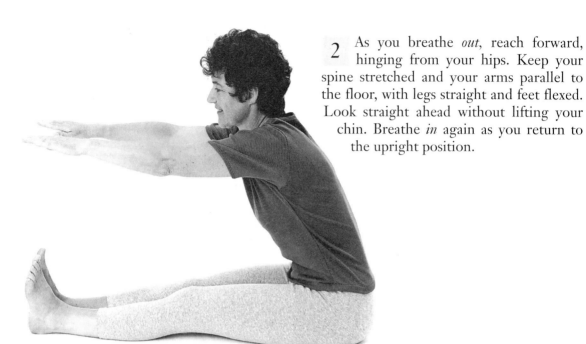

2 As you breathe *out*, reach forward, hinging from your hips. Keep your spine stretched and your arms parallel to the floor, with legs straight and feet flexed. Look straight ahead without lifting your chin. Breathe *in* again as you return to the upright position.

3 Breathe *out* as you lean backwards, hinging from your hips and keeping arms parallel to the floor, legs straight and feet flexed. Keep your spine stretched, while leaning back as far as you can. Keep your legs against the floor. Breathe *in* to come back to the upright position. Repeat the sequence until you feel that you have thoroughly worked the lower abdominal muscles.

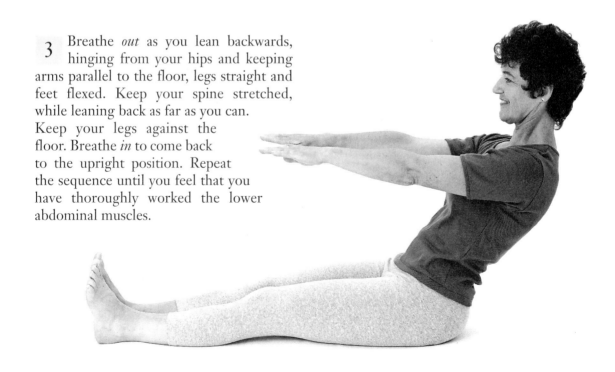

THIGH GRIP

1 Bend your knees and bring your feet close to your buttocks, so that you can wrap your arms around the backs of your thighs and squeeze your legs against your chest – sitting up as straight as you can. Breathe *in* and stretch the spine *up*.

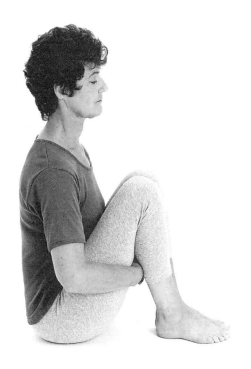

2 As you breathe *out*, slowly slide your feet away from you, maintaining contact between your thighs and your chest as you inch forward. Stop when you need to breathe *in* and concentrate on straightening the spine and keeping your head in line. Do not let your chin poke forward. As you breathe *out*, walk your feet forward a little more.

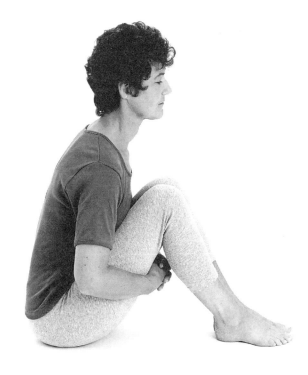

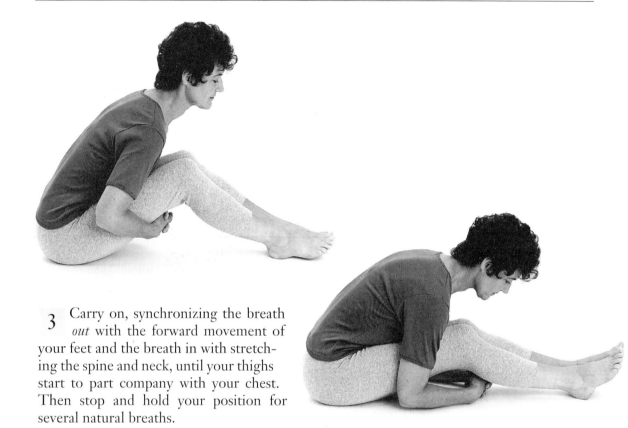

3 Carry on, synchronizing the breath *out* with the forward movement of your feet and the breath in with stretching the spine and neck, until your thighs start to part company with your chest. Then stop and hold your position for several natural breaths.

FORWARD BEND

When (or if!) your legs become almost straight in Step 3 of the Thigh Grip, you can remove your arms from underneath them and settle into the classical position – head on shins, elbows either side of straight legs, forearms resting on the floor, and palms near the feet, turned upwards. Stay in this position with slow natural breathing until you feel strain (ragged breathing, shaky limbs or difficulty in holding the pose).

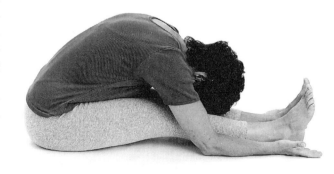

BACK ARCHING RELEASE

Come out of the Forward Bend position very gently and sit for a moment in Dandasana. You may feel like stretching the spine the opposite way, as a 'counterpose' to your forward bend.

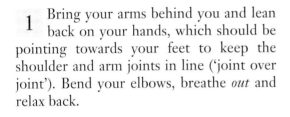

1 Bring your arms behind you and lean back on your hands, which should be pointing towards your feet to keep the shoulder and arm joints in line ('joint over joint'). Bend your elbows, breathe *out* and relax back.

2 As you breathe *in*, straighten your arms, arch your back and push your sternum (breastbone) up as high as you can, to stretch the front of your body.

Repeat a few times, slowly and with awareness of how your body is feeling.

FINGER WALKING

This is a strong sequence which loosens and opens the hips and stretches the inner thigh and buttock muscles. Take it gently! In our western way of life we do not often spread the legs wide or squat down on the floor. We sit, stand and walk with our legs close together. As a result we are apt to suffer from trouble in the hip joints later in life. This sequence can ease or prevent stiffness in the hips, which may feel very inflexible when you first attempt these exercises. With a little persistent but gentle practice you will soon see a vast improvement!

Finger Walking is an excellent preparation for Siddhasana, the classical seated pose used for breathing and meditation (see Chapter 13).

1 Start with a good, upward-stretched Dandasana. Spread your legs as wide apart as they will go, keeping your spine erect. Keep your legs straight and your feet flexed, toes up – stretching the hamstring muscles again! Too much sitting shortens them; so does standing and walking in high heels. Keep both your buttocks in contact with the floor all the time.

Place both hands on the floor in front of you and breathe *in*, stretching *up*. As you start to breathe *out*, 'walk' your fingers forward along the floor, bending the body from the hips. Stop and stretch the spine *up* as you breathe *in* and continue 'walking' your fingers forward as you breathe *out*.

Repeat until you have got as far as you can reach, then stop and hold the position with natural breathing. You should feel your tight muscles relaxing, 'paying out' each time you breathe *out*. When you have held this position long enough, gently 'walk' your fingers back again. Repeat if you feel like it.

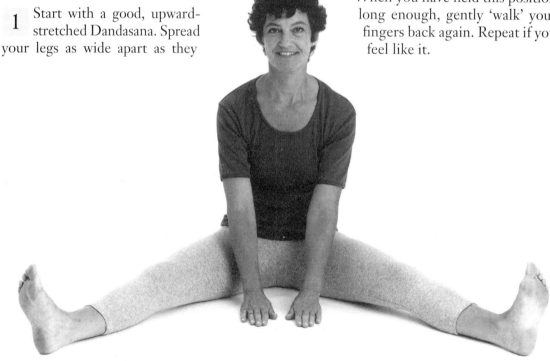

2 Now place one hand each side of your right leg and 'walk' your fingers along the floor towards your flexed foot, as you breathe *out*. Remember to keep your back straight and your left foot flexed, with your left buttock on the floor! Hold the position as you breathe *in* and 'walk' further as you breathe *out*. Repeat until you can reach no further without lifting your left buttock. Stop there and hold, with natural breathing. 'Walk' your fingers back very gently when you are ready.

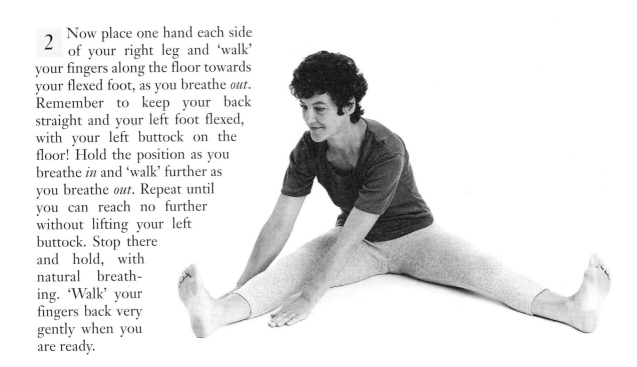

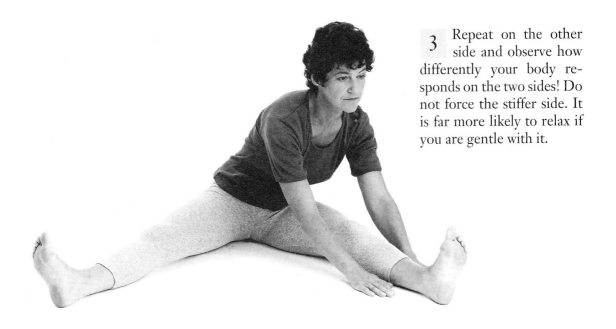

3 Repeat on the other side and observe how differently your body responds on the two sides! Do not force the stiffer side. It is far more likely to relax if you are gentle with it.

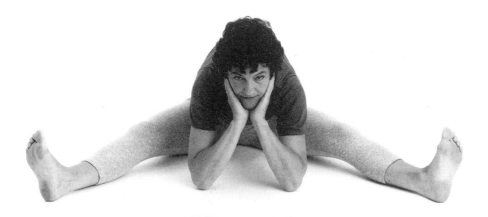

The positions shown here, resting the chin in the hands with elbows on the floor, will probably only be possible after considerable practice of the preceding stages. However, some people do loosen up very easily! Listen to your body and respect what it tells you. The wider apart your legs are, the nearer your chin will be to the floor. Keep your mind in all of your body – legs straight, feet flexed, buttocks on the floor.

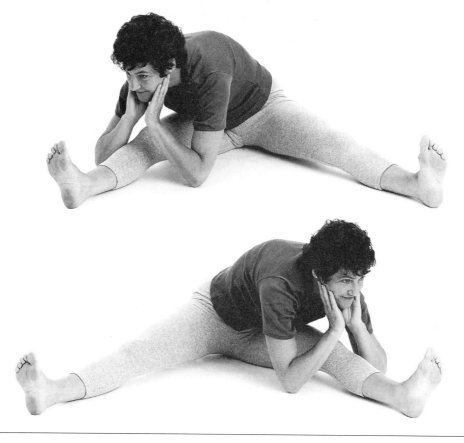

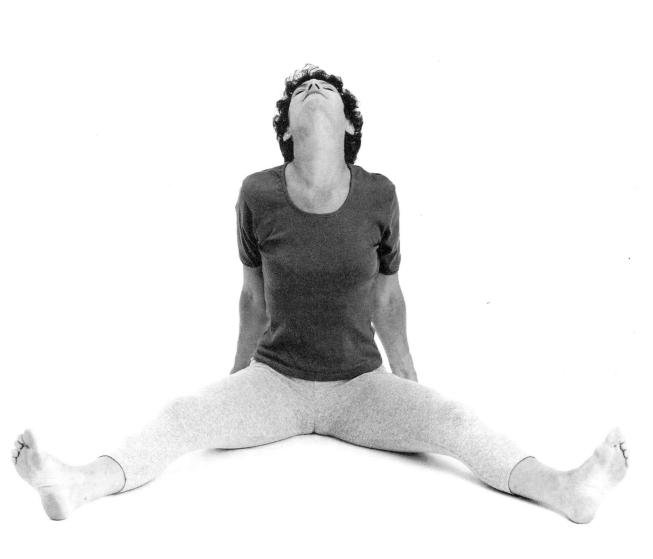

Yoga is always concerned with the whole body, plus the breathing, plus focus, plus a relaxed and peaceful attitude. Stressful effort does not produce yoga, it only produces gymnastics!

When you have finished all the Finger Walking you want to do, sit up very gently and rest on your hands, placed on the floor behind you for support. Observe how you are feeling.

BACK ARCHING RELEASE VARIATION

You may want to do the Back Arching Release (see page 47) shown after the classical forward bend, or this variation.

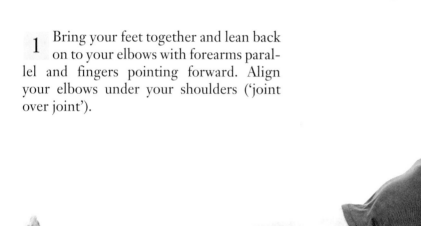

1 Bring your feet together and lean back on to your elbows with forearms parallel and fingers pointing forward. Align your elbows under your shoulders ('joint over joint').

2 Relax as you breathe *out* and lift the sternum (breastbone), arching the back, as you breathe *in*. Repeat until your body feels comfortable and restored after the strenuous forward-bending exercises.

It is also sometimes useful to do the Back Arching Release before you start any forward-bending sequences. Remember to use it always after any prolonged forward-bending activity, such as gardening.

CHAPTER 7

GRACEFUL MOVEMENT

Working shoulders and arms

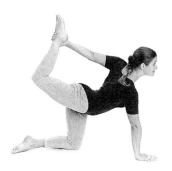

THE PREVIOUS CHAPTER introduced sequences that stretch the lower half of the body. The upper half also needs limbering. The pectoral muscles across the chest often become tight as a result of habitual poor posture, which rounds the shoulders and narrows the chest. Nervous tension around the neck, shoulders and upper arms also causes tightness in the muscles which can be released by stretching movements.

The arms and hands are toned and strengthened through supporting the body's weight. This counteracts the weakening effect of carrying heavy items, such as shopping bags or briefcases, which pull the shoulders downwards and out of position. The sequences following all start from Vajrasana.

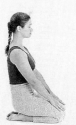

STARTING POSITION

Kneel in Vajrasana (see Chapter 3 for detailed instructions). The support here is provided by the folded legs, with the spine stretching up from this base. Get into a settled position and watch your breathing for a few minutes.

KNEELING STRETCH

1 As you breathe *out*, crawl your fingers along the floor, keeping your buttocks on your heels, if possible. Pause to stretch up in the spine as you breathe *in*. Crawl forward some more as you breathe *out*.

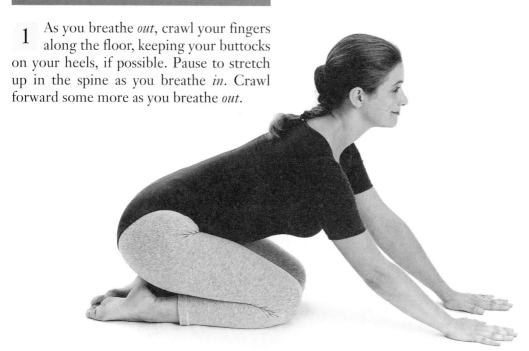

2 Repeat until you are fully stretched, then (breathing naturally) stretch out your fingers as though you were hanging on to a cliff and reach even further forward. This is a wonderfully 'restoring' pose, which realigns the spine after any activity that compresses it, such as prolonged driving, sitting or carrying heavy objects.

DIAMOND STRETCH

This is a variation of the Kneeling Stretch which also stretches in the hips and accommodates a large abdomen, as in pregnancy.

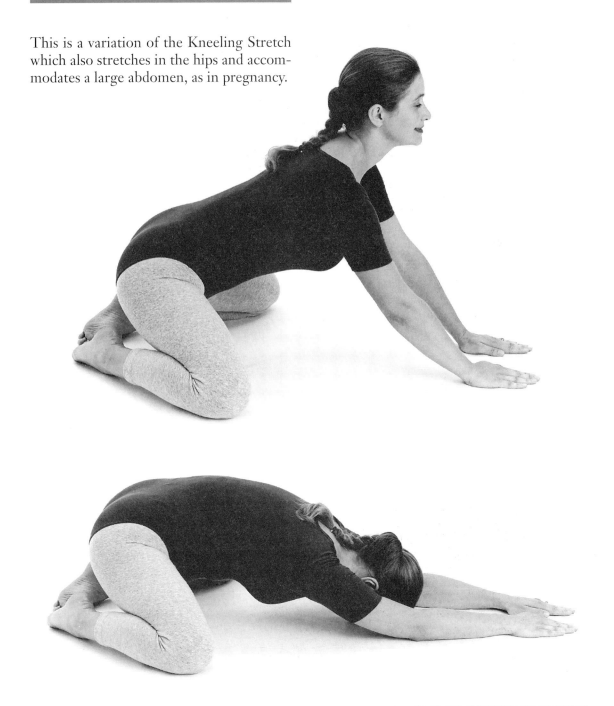

FROG

Resting the elbows on the floor and the head in the hands is a very comfortable variation for many people.

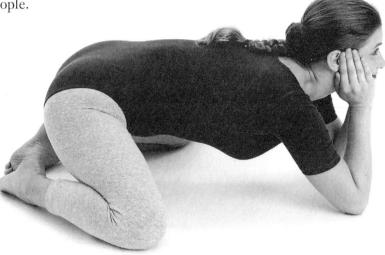

CHILD

From Kneeling Stretch, once the spine is fully extended, bring your arms around and hold your feet, if you can reach. Keep your buttocks on your heels!

It is often helpful to go into one of the above postures if you feel in need of a rest between sequences.

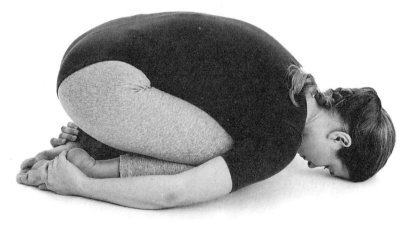

CAT STRETCH

1 From Kneeling Stretch, lift your buttocks up from your heels and bring your weight forward on to your hands, which are already stretched out and shoulder-width apart ('joint over joint' to take your weight safely). Bring your knees hip-width apart ('joint over joint') and kneel four-square with straight spine and neck. Take time to adjust your position, so that your spine feels neither over-stretched nor compressed, and your weight is evenly balanced.

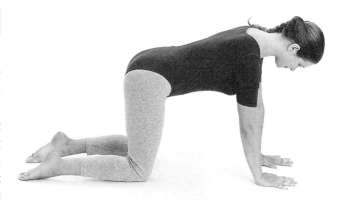

> WATCHPOINT: Keep your arms straight throughout!

2 As you breathe *in*, pull your waist down towards the floor and look *up* at the ceiling, stretching all of the front of your body.

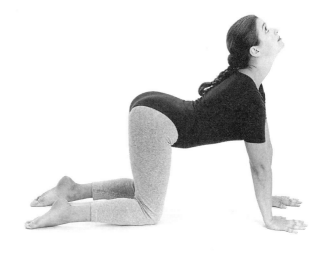

3 As you breathe *out*, pull your waist up towards the ceiling and look *down*, with your head tucked between your straight arms, at your navel. This stretches all the back of your body. This is a good sequence for visualization. Imagine light travelling *up* your spine as you breathe *in* and *down* as you breathe *out*.

Repeat these movements in a gentle flowing manner, synchronized with your breathing, until you feel you have loosened up your whole spine, including your neck. The Cat Stretch brings great awareness to the spine, and also flexibility. Return to Kneeling Stretch.

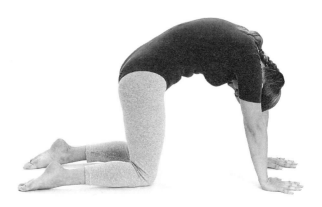

TIGER STRETCH

From the Cat Stretch position, raise your opposite arm and leg and stretch them out horizontally. Take care that your arm comes forward and your leg goes back – not veering to the side! Balance for a while, then return to the starting position and repeat with your other arm and leg. You can also experiment with raising an arm and a leg on the same side. This is a fine balance and a good stretch.

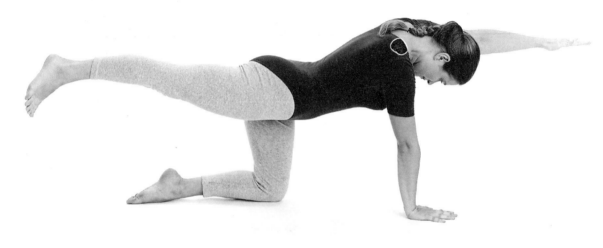

TIGER BOW

From the Tiger Stretch you can go on to raise your extended foot as high as possible, bending your knee. Hold on to your foot with your outstretched hand, bringing your arm behind you. Move slowly, to maintain your balance. Look *up* and reach *up* with your joined foot and hand. Balance for a while, then return to the starting position and repeat with your other arm and leg. The Tiger Bow can also be done with both arm and leg raised on the same side.

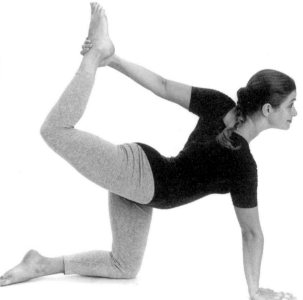

WATCHPOINT: Make certain that you are working in bare feet on a non-slip surface for all the positions that follow.

DOG

1 From the Cat Stretch position, lift your heels and tuck your toes under.

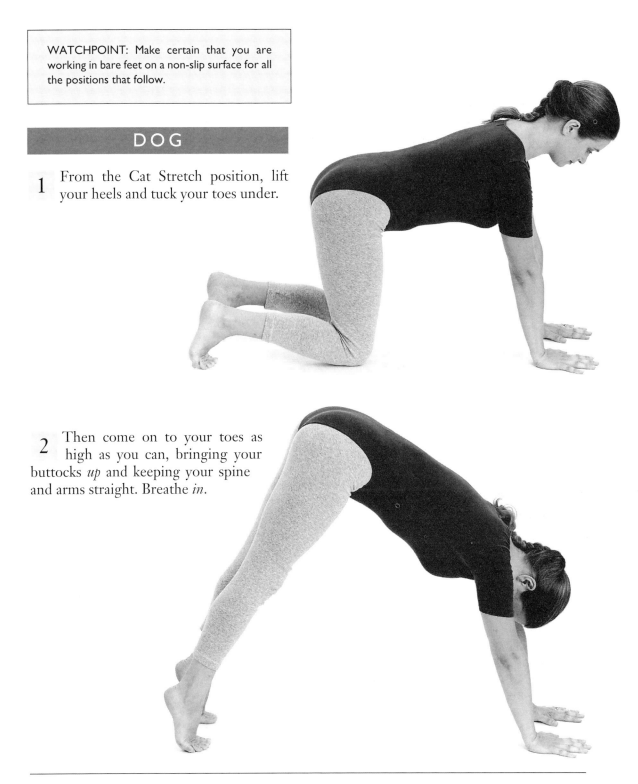

2 Then come on to your toes as high as you can, bringing your buttocks *up* and keeping your spine and arms straight. Breathe *in*.

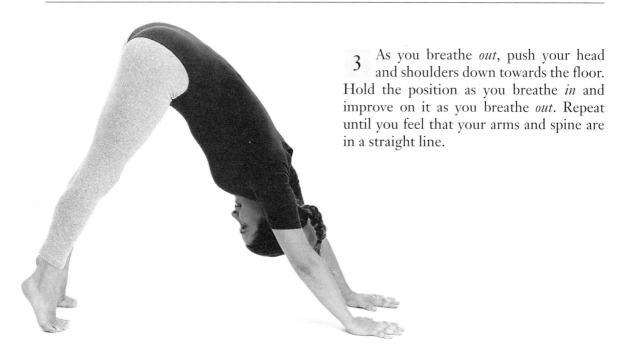

3 As you breathe *out*, push your head and shoulders down towards the floor. Hold the position as you breathe *in* and improve on it as you breathe *out*. Repeat until you feel that your arms and spine are in a straight line.

4 Then start working to get your heels down on to the floor. This will stretch the hamstring muscles at the backs of your legs. It may help to lower one heel at a time in a rhythmic 'dance' synchronized with your breathing. Keep also pushing the crown of your head towards the floor.

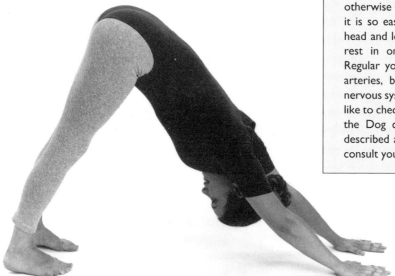

WATCHPOINT: The Dog is an inverted position, where your head is lower than your heart. Do not stay in it if you feel the blood rushing to your head, your heart 'banging' or your breath getting 'ragged'. These may be signs of strain in the cardio-vascular system. The Dog is a good test of the health – or otherwise – of the heart and arteries, because it is so easy to get out of! Simply raise your head and lower your knees to the floor, then rest in one of the positions given above. Regular yoga practice benefits the heart and arteries, because it balances the autonomic nervous system and relieves stress. So you may like to check from time to time whether or not the Dog causes you any of the discomfort described above. If it does, it may be wise to consult your doctor.

PLANK

This is part of a vigorous, dynamic sequence that combines many of the movements given above. From the Dog, take your weight forward on to your hands as you breathe *in*, so that your body is in a straight line. It is helpful to get a friend to check, as we are less aware of our backs than our fronts! As you breathe *out*, return to the Dog position – or to the Side Plank shown below.

SIDE PLANK

From the Plank, turn your whole body to one side and lean your weight on one arm and one foot only, as you breathe *out*. Smile! As you breathe *in*, return to the Plank, then repeat the Side Plank on the other side, as you breathe *out*.

THE WHOLE SEQUENCE

Start in Vajrasana.

Breathe *out* as you move into the Kneeling Stretch.

Breathe *in* as you move into the Cat Stretch.

Breathe *out* as you move into the Dog.

Breathe *in* as you move into the Plank.

Breathe *out* as you move into the Side Plank.

Breathe *in* as you return to the Dog.

Breathe *out* as you move into the Side Plank on the other side.

Breathe *in* as you return to the Plank.

Breathe *out* as you return to the Dog.

Breathe *in* as you return to the Cat Stretch.

Breathe *out* as you return to the Kneeling Stretch.

Breathe *in* as you return to the Vajrasana.

Repeat the sequence, or rest in the Diamond Stretch, Frog or Child.

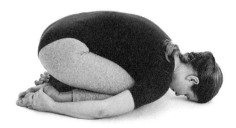

CHAPTER 8

STANDING WARM-UPS

For strength and vitality

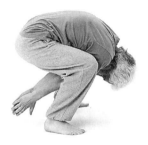

THE SEQUENCES IN this chapter really get the blood moving and the energy going! Yoga can do wonders for the spine – as long as you practise self-awareness and relaxation as well as the physical movements. You swing through the following movements as you synchronize them with your breathing. Enjoy the sense of release and physical wellbeing that vigorous activity can bring!

At the same time, remember to stay centred and relaxed. If any of the movements seem difficult, simply slow them down, allowing more time for the body to adjust as it leaves one position and enters another. Stop and rest whenever you feel the need, focusing on breathing *out slowly*.

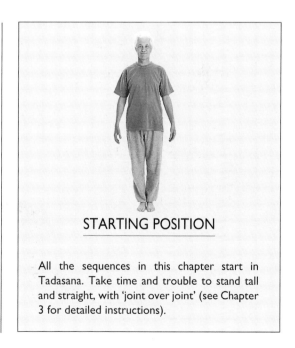

STARTING POSITION

All the sequences in this chapter start in Tadasana. Take time and trouble to stand tall and straight, with 'joint over joint' (see Chapter 3 for detailed instructions).

SQUATS

1 Bring your feet 60–90 cm (2–3 ft) apart, with your toes turned outwards about 45 degrees. This is to ensure that when you bend your knees outwards – they will be aligned directly over your ankles and feet ('joint over joint'). Adjust your position until you can bend your knees comfortably and keep your insteps raised. The weight should always be on the outsides of the feet, with the ankles over the heels – not falling inwards and causing the arches to drop.

It may take some practice to strengthen and align your ankles and feet, so that they remain firmly in place while you bend your knees.

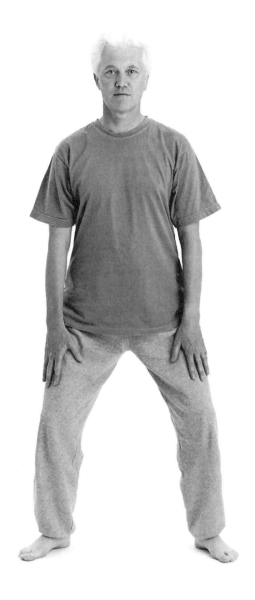

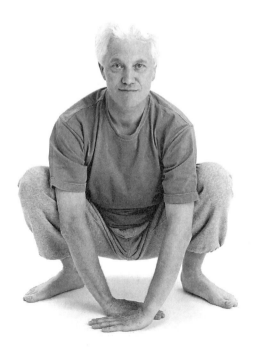

2 Bend your knees deeply, putting your hands on the floor in front of you with your wrists under your elbows and your thumbs towards your body. Let your hands take most of your weight, while you work to align your knees, ankles and feet.

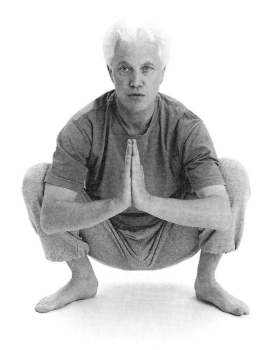

3 When you are ready, bring your hands into the 'Indian greeting' position, thumbs to heart. Press your palms together and use your elbows to push out against your inner thighs. This leverage to the side will stretch your inner thigh muscles, improve the alignment of your legs and allow you to squat down even more. As you breathe *in*, push against your thighs, arch your back and look *up*. As you breathe *out*, relax and sink down lower.

Repeat these movements, synchronized to your breathing, until you feel that your lower back, hips and legs have loosened up.

> WATCHPOINT: The next movement will invert the body, with your head lower than your heart. Please note the precautions given for the Dog pose in Chapter 7. If you feel at all uncomfortable upside down, simply return to the Squats position.

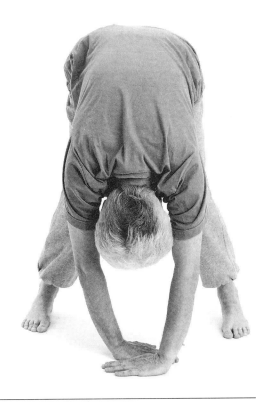

4 As you breathe *out*, bring your hands back to the floor as before and slowly straighten your legs, bringing you into a standing forward bend. As you breathe *in*, bend your knees and squat down again, leaving your hands on the floor.

Repeat these movements, synchronized with the breath, to stretch the lower back and the hamstring muscles at the back of your legs. If you wish, you can alternate with some more pushing movements, bringing the hands back to the 'Indian greeting' position.

SKIING

This is a dynamic sequence that wakes up and loosens the legs, arms and spine.

1 Stand tall in Tadasana. Then separate your feet to hip-width apart, with toes pointing forward and arches lifted ('joint over joint' so that you can bend your knees safely). Breathing *in*, raise your arms and swing them up high in front of you, leaning back with knees bent.

WATCHPOINT: Keep the knees bent all the time, to protect the lower back. If you are inclined to have lower back pain, you may prefer not to practise the Skiing or the Woodchopper sequences for the time being. Continue to do plenty of twisting movements lying down (See Chapter 5) to make the spine more flexible. The Jackknife (see Chapter 6) loosens the lower back and strengthens the abdominal muscles, while the Kneeling Stretch (see Chapter 7) lengthens the spine and removes painful compression.

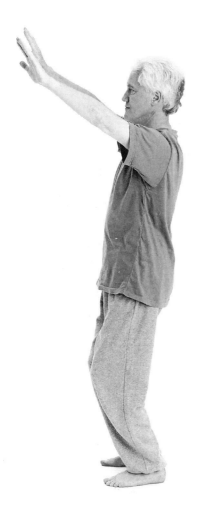

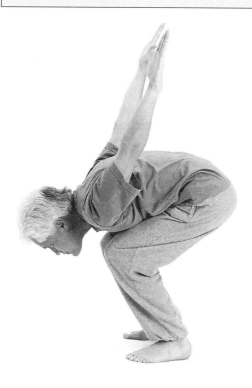

2 Breathing *out* vigorously, sweep your arms forward, down and back as high as you can. At the same time, bend your knees as deeply as possible, keeping your knees and feet in line. They may be inclined to splay out to the side if you let your arches drop.

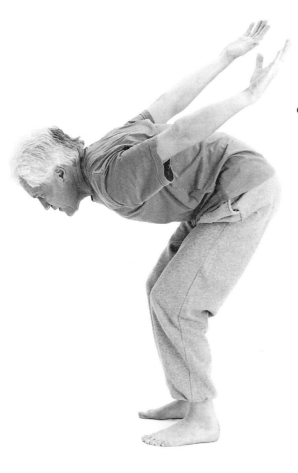

You may find that bending halfway down is enough for the time being.

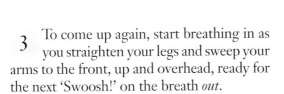

3 To come up again, start breathing in as you straighten your legs and sweep your arms to the front, up and overhead, ready for the next 'Swoosh!' on the breath *out*.

Repeat until you feel invigorated and loosened up.

WOODCHOPPER

This is similar to Skiing, but more dynamic, especially the breathing.

1 Stand in Tadasana. Have your feet about 75 cm (30 in) apart, wide enough to be able to swing your hands, arms and trunk between your legs. Your feet should point to the front, arches lifted ('joint over joint'). Place your hands in the 'Indian greeting' position, palms together throughout. Bring them forward and up and back in a wide sweep, keeping your knees bent, as you breathe *in* deeply.

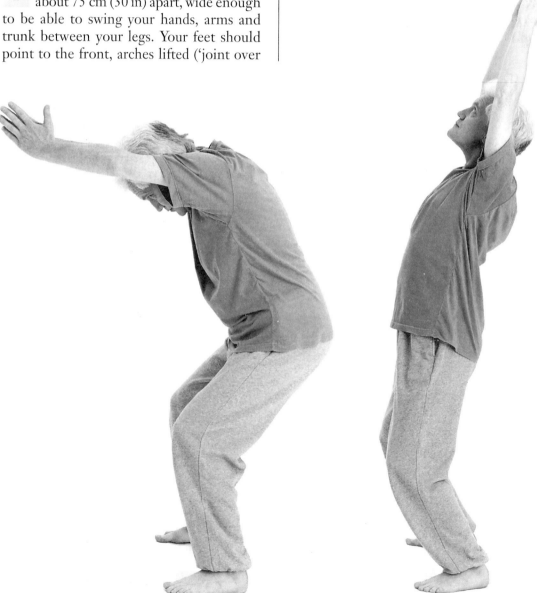

2 Breathe *out* through your mouth, making a loud 'Haah!' sound and expelling as much air as possible while you take your hands and arms down between your legs and out behind you. Keep your knees deeply bent and take care not to catch your fingers on the floor as you sweep them through!

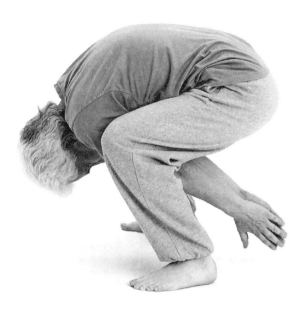

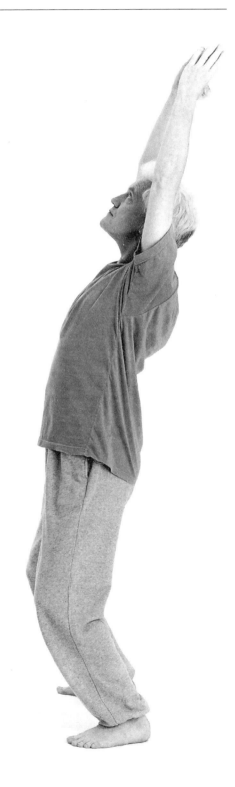

Bring your arms up and back again as you breathe *in* through your nose and repeat the 'Haah!' as you breathe *out* through your mouth, swinging your arms down and through.

Repeat several times. This type of breathing is very invigorating because it clears the lungs of stale air.

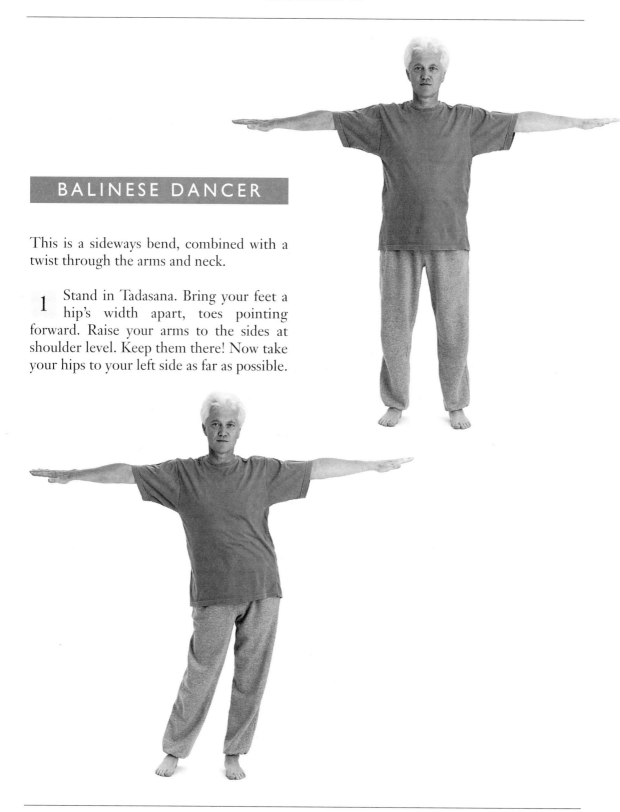

BALINESE DANCER

This is a sideways bend, combined with a twist through the arms and neck.

1   Stand in Tadasana. Bring your feet a hip's width apart, toes pointing forward. Raise your arms to the sides at shoulder level. Keep them there! Now take your hips to your left side as far as possible.

2 Turn your right palm *up* and your left palm *down* and round to face behind you. Stretch into your fingertips. You will feel this stretch along both arms and through your shoulders – like twisting a rope. Turn your head to look at your right palm. Straighten up again and repeat these movements to the other side.

When you have got your movements co-ordinated, add the breathing. Breathe *in* as you stand tall, facing front. Breathe *out* as you move the hips to the side, 'twist the rope' and turn your head to face your upturned palm. Breathe *in* as you 'undo' the pose and stand tall again, facing front. Breathe *out* as you repeat to the other side.

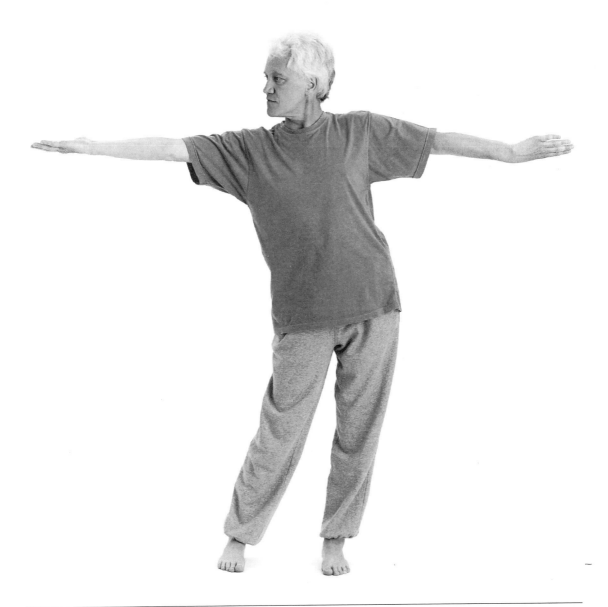

Once you get into a rhythm, this is a beautiful, graceful movement which relieves tension in the hips, shoulders, arms and neck. Repeat several times. Keep your arms up at shoulder level all the time!

3 When you are ready to come out of the Balinese Dancer pose, stretch across your shoulders and along your arms to your fingertips. Then lower your hands very, very slowly.

Let tension 'drip' from your fingertips, as you let go of all those burdens you have been shouldering for so long! Take a minute or so to lower your arms. You will feel wonderful afterwards.

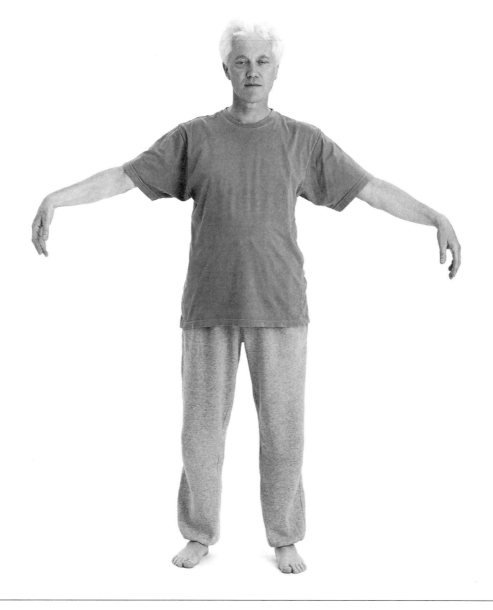

PART THREE

SPECIFIC AREAS

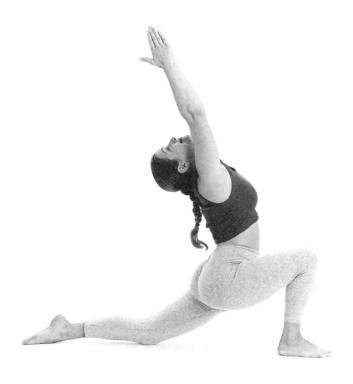

CHAPTER 9

LEGS AND LOWER BACK

Building a strong foundation

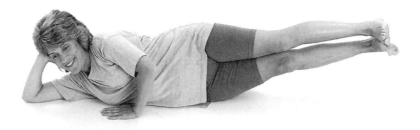

YOGA WORKS ON the whole body-mind, even if one part of the body is stretched more than other parts. The whole person is always involved, with movement and breath 'yoked' to mental concentration and relaxation. It therefore makes good sense to practise a wide variety of postures and sequences, rather than sticking to a few that are targeted to your personal problem areas. The limbering sequences shown in the previous chapters will strengthen and loosen you up all over. First practise one or two from each chapter, ringing the changes to get as much variety as possible, and then you will be ready to work on specific areas.

Below are exercises that strengthen the muscles of the legs, abdomen, buttocks and lower back. This toning will also improve your silhouette.

Extra preparation for this series may be needed, in addition to overall limbering. This will depend on your personal areas of weakness and strength. Forehead to Knee and Knees to Chest (see Chapter 5) work the spine, legs and abdominal muscles. So does the Jackknife (see Chapter 6). Finger Walking (see Chapter 6) loosens the muscles around the hip joints, to help you with the sideways leg lift. Practise all the above to gain strength and confidence before you start on this section.

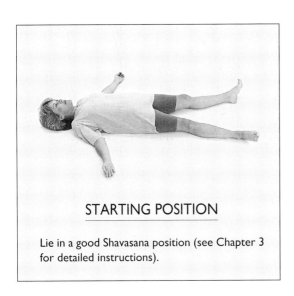

STARTING POSITION

Lie in a good Shavasana position (see Chapter 3 for detailed instructions).

ONE-LEG CYCLING

This movement works stongly on the lower abdominal muscles which help to hold the lower back in proper alignment. If these muscles are weak, they allow the strong back muscles to over-contract. Muscles work in pairs, pulling against each other to provide the correct tension. That is how we are able to stand upright. If one side of the pair fails, the other pulls too tightly – as is sometimes visible in the face of a person who has suffered a stroke.

Bring your legs together and place your arms alongside your body for support, with the palms facing down and pressing against the floor. This position gives support to your back which is essential.

WATCHPOINT: Legs are extremely heavy. You want your abdominal muscles to contract to do the lifting, supported by your arms. Your spine should not be involved at all. To ensure that the spine remains passive, tuck your chin down and lengthen your neck. Press your waist into the floor and keep your coccyx (tailbone) against the floor by tilting your pelvis slightly. Press down on your palms.

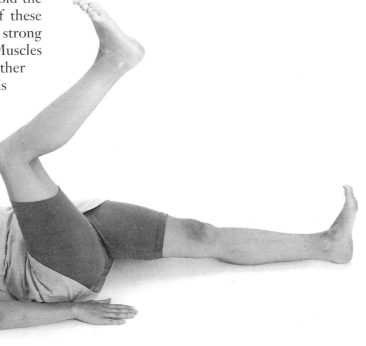

When you are in position, bend your right knee, keeping your left leg straight with foot flexed and toes pointing to the ceiling. Raise your right leg and draw large circles in the air with it, as though you were cycling. Gradually make the circles larger and larger. Keep your back flat on the floor! After a while bring your right leg down to the floor, with knee bent, and rest. Then lift it again and cycle backwards for a while, making your circles larger and larger.

When you have finished, rest in Shavasana for a moment and observe how you have been tightening the lower abdominal muscles. Check that your back still feels relaxed and is flat on the floor. Then repeat the sequence, cycling forwards and backwards with your left leg.

STRANDED BEETLE

Keeping your back flat and relaxed, bend both knees and hold them in your palms. Make sure your coccyx (tailbone) is pressed to the floor and your chin is tucked down. Allow your legs to relax, supported in your cupped palms. Then gently rotate both legs from the hips, in opposite directions – out and in towards each other. You will feel your abdominal and lower back muscles 'melt' into the floor.

This simple exercise is marvellous for relieving a sore and aching back at any time. It can also be a great help if you are prone to sciatica. This is often caused by tight muscles pulling the spine out of alignment, to press on the nerve that travels down your leg.

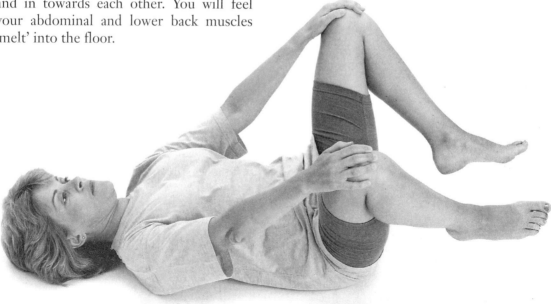

SIDE SNAKE

The weight of your leg is used here to strengthen the muscles at the side of your body, which are also involved in standing upright. It is a little like supporting a heavy pillar with guide ropes!

1 Keeping the straight line of the Shavasana position, roll on to your right side with both arms in line above your head, palms together. Avoid rolling backwards! Your right shoulder and hip should press into the floor. Flex both your feet. This will help you to balance.

> WATCHPOINT: Keep in a straight line! After a few repetitions you will probably find yourself in the boomerang position, with feet and hands jutting forward. Check and adjust frequently!

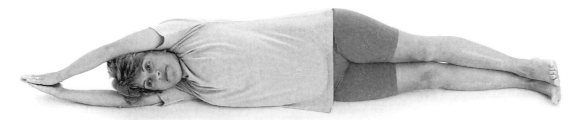

2 As you breathe *in*, raise your left arm and left leg until they meet. Keep your feet flexed, the right foot to balance you and the left to work your leg muscles.

As you breathe *out*, lower your left hand to clap the palm of your right hand loudly and your left leg to lie over your right leg. You can shout 'Haah!' at the same time, if you like, to clear stale air from your lungs.

Repeat these movements several times; then roll into Shavasana and get into position on your left side. Repeat the same number of times on this side.

> WATCHPOINT: Your raised leg should not jut forward. To work in your hip joint, lift it *up*, in line with your body, like a pair of scissors.

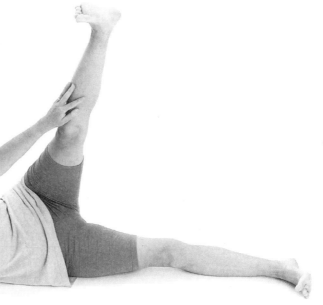

SIDE LOCUST

1 Lie on your right elbow, with your head cupped in your right hand. As with the Side Snake above, keep adjusting so that you are in a straight line from elbow to feet. Keep both feet flexed. To help you to balance, place your left palm on the floor in front of your sternum (breastbone), fingers pointing towards your head. Roll a little forward on to this hand to keep your line as you breathe *in* and raise your left leg. Hold this position, with natural breathing, for as long as you comfortably can.

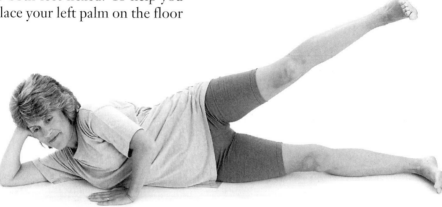

2 Lower your leg and rest for a moment, before breathing *in* to raise both legs and holding them up for as long as you can. When you have held the position long enough, lower your legs and roll into Shavasana. Rest for a moment before repeating on the other side. You may find that one side of your body seems much stronger than the other. This is quite natural. We are all unbalanced in many ways! Yoga is always concerned with achieving balance and harmony. It teaches us awareness and acceptance of both our weaknesses and strengths.

WATCHPOINT: Feel as though you are raising your leg, or legs, up behind you – to 'open' the front of the body and avoid the boomerang effect.

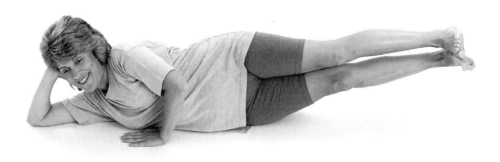

EXTENDED STANDING FORWARD BEND

WATCHPOINT: This is an inverted pose, which you may want to stay in for several minutes. Please read the comments on inverted poses in Chapter 7 again.

The following posture works strongly in the lower back, loosening any tightness at the sides (with the wide-legged position) as well as at the back (with the forward-bending position). Suitable preparation, in addition to general limbering, would be the Dog (see Chapter 7), Knee Rolls (see Chapter 5), Finger Walking (see Chapter 6), the Diamond Stretch (see Chapter 7), Squats (see Chapter 8) and Skiing (see Chapter 8).

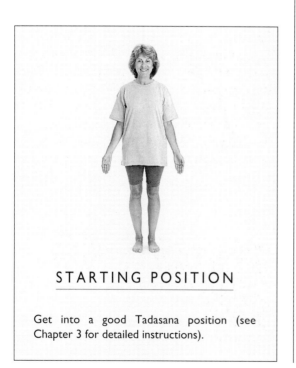

STARTING POSITION

Get into a good Tadasana position (see Chapter 3 for detailed instructions).

1 From Tadasana, spread your legs as wide apart as possible. Turn your heels out, to get a firm grip on the floor with the outsides of your feet. Keep your insteps raised and strong. Work on your feet and ankles for a while, before bending forward.

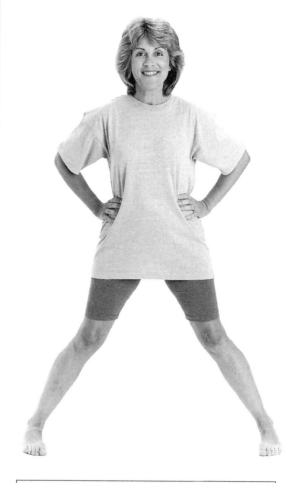

WATCHPOINT: Make sure that you are working in bare feet and on a non-slip surface. Pulling a muscle in the groin, due to slipping, can be very painful and take a long time to heal!

2 When you feel balanced, with your feet firmly 'rooted' and as far apart as possible, heels out, bend forward from the hips. Keeping your legs straight throughout, bring your hands to the floor. Aim to bring your wrists and palms back in line with your ankles and feet, bending your elbows. Hold this position, breathing naturally, until you feel yourself weakening. Come out of it, 'walking' your fingers forward, before you lose control in your feet and legs.

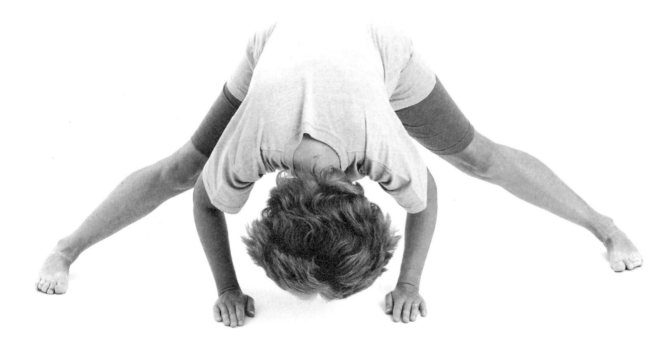

Repeat once, trying to improve your position. You may find that you are able to place the crown of your head on the floor, in line between your wrists, if you are supple enough in your hips.

When you have finished, return slowly to Tadasana and quietly observe how you feel, before allowing your body to choose its own position to relax in – maybe a gentle Squat, a Stranded Beetle or Shavasana.

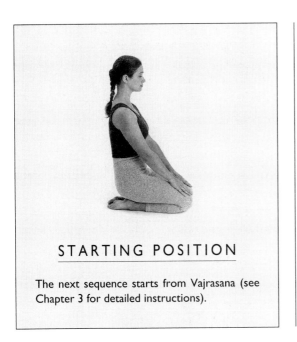

STARTING POSITION

The next sequence starts from Vajrasana (see Chapter 3 for detailed instructions).

CAT STRETCH

This sequence is aimed at strengthening the muscles in the abdomen, buttocks and legs. It also works strongly on the muscles around the hip joints, as the leg is lifted to the side in different positions, and on the upper back and arms. It may seem hard to begin with, but quickly gets easier with practice as the muscles gain in tone. A good preparation would be the Dog–Cat Stretch–Plank sequence in Chapter 7, which uses many of the same positions.

From a good Vajrasana position stretch forward into the Kneeling Stretch and rise up from there into the Cat Stretch (see Chapter 7 for detailed instructions).

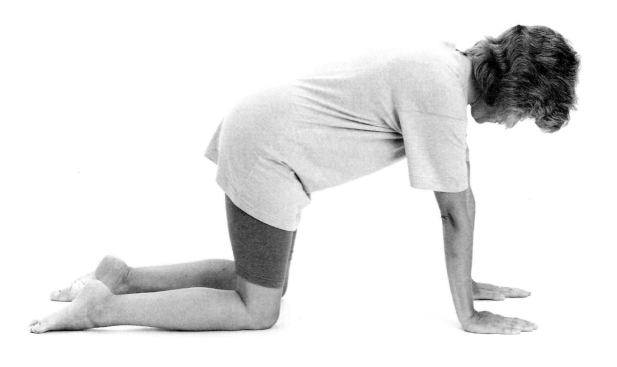

ROVER'S REVENGE

1 Keeping the whole body steady and in line, as in the Cat Stretch above, raise your right knee to the side, to hip level, as you breathe *in* – without changing its position. The only movement should be in the hip joint.

Lower your knee to the floor as you breathe *out*. Repeat this movement about six times, then repeat on the other side, raising and lowering your left knee.

WATCHPOINT: The spine, head and neck should remain in line, regardless of what your leg is doing! Keep your arms straight throughout. The leg that is being raised should come up to the side and slightly forward of the other knee, to counteract the tendency to take it back. If you do raise your leg when badly aligned (twisted or behind you), you may get a cramp in the hips or buttocks, through pinching a nerve. Should this happen, roll on to your back into the Stranded Beetle to ease the hip joints. The cramp will soon pass!

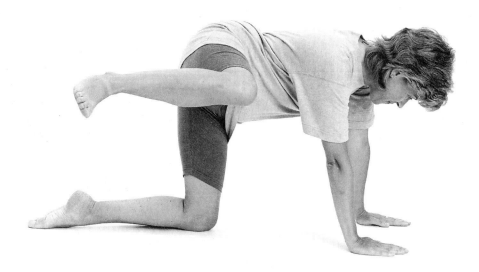

You may find that this movement is much easier on one side than the other. This is quite natural. It will, in any case, get easier with practice. Working more times on the weak side will strengthen it.

2 Stretch your right leg out to the side, with your right heel slightly forward of your left knee and your right foot flexed.

Keep everything else steady and in line as you breathe *in* and raise your straight right leg up to hip level. If this is impossible, raise it as high as you can! Lower it to the floor, still in line, as you breathe *out*.

Repeat about six times, then repeat the sequence on the other side, raising your straight left leg. Again, one side may be much stronger than the other.

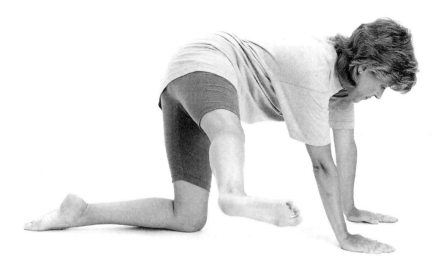

3 Now stretch your right leg out to the side, with the heel slightly forward of the left knee, and rotate the whole leg in the hip joint so that the sole of your right foot faces the floor. When you are ready, breathe *in* and lift your leg straight up – if you can! – as high as you can. Notice how the front thigh muscles tighten. Lower as you breathe *out*. If this is easy for you, repeat the movement a few times with the right leg, then the same number of times with the left leg.

When you have finished, hold the Cat Stretch position for a moment, observing how you feel. Then allow your body to choose its preferred resting position – perhaps the Child or Frog (see Chapter 7), Shavasana, or maybe something else.

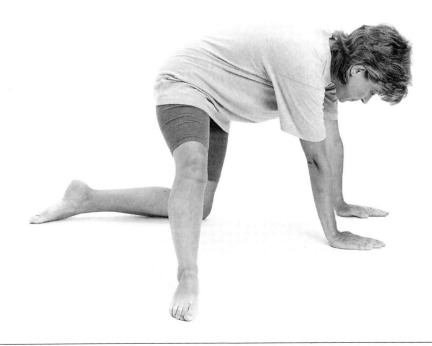

CHAPTER 10

EASING THE HIPS AND PELVIS

For flexibility and grace

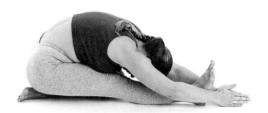

THE FOLLOWING SEQUENCES, while stretching the arms and shoulders and spine, also work strongly in the hips and legs – as you will discover!

You should work towards a feeling of being lengthened through the middle, so that your ribs and chest lift up and away from the abdomen and pelvis. In daily life it is so easy to succumb to the combined effects of gravity and fatigue, so that you collapse around the middle. This restricts the natural freedom of the diaphragm to pump air in and out of your lungs – resulting in further fatigue through inadequate breathing. Stretch up and out of this vicious cycle!

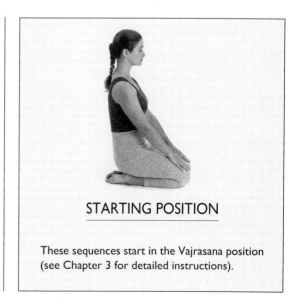

STARTING POSITION

These sequences start in the Vajrasana position (see Chapter 3 for detailed instructions).

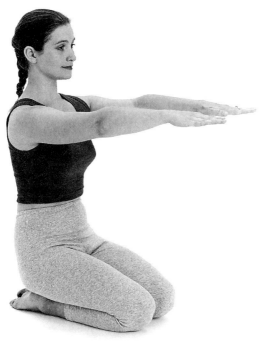

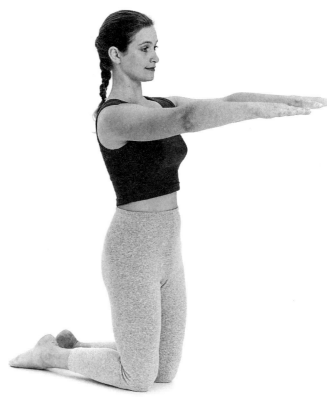

HIP SWINGS

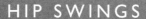

1 From the Vajrasana position, raise your arms up in front of you at shoulder height, keeping them parallel all the time. Rise up on to your knees as you breathe *in*, stretching up through your spine.

2 Sit on the floor to the left of your feet as you breathe *out*, twisting at the waist to bring your chest and arms round to the right, looking as far round behind you as you can. As you breathe *in*, kneel up again and look forward. Repeat, breathing *out* as you sit on the right side of your feet and twist to the left. Continue this sequence and feel yourself stretching and loosening up all over, until you are ready to move on to the next step.

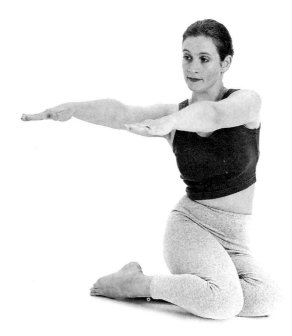

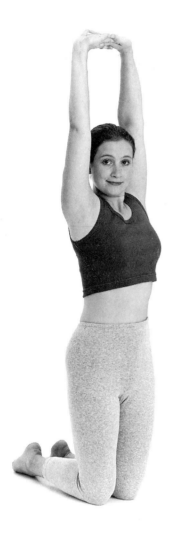

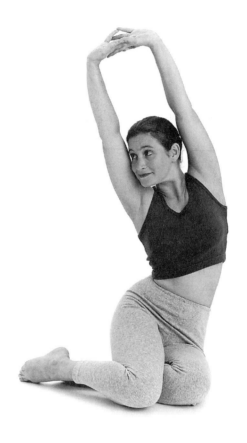

3   This time, as you breathe *in*, kneel up and take your hands overhead, clasping them together with the palms facing upwards. Stretch fully through the chest and arms. As you breathe *out*, sit on the floor to the left of your feet, and twist the upper body round to look behind you to the right. Breathe *in* to rise again to your knees, and *out* to sit on the right side of your feet and twist to the left. Repeat this sequence until you feel tired, then rest in the Child (see page 56) to relax your arms.

WATCHPOINT: Be sure to keep the upward stretch throughout, so that your arms stretch up beside your ears and your hands are directly above your erect head. This may take some practice but, as with all yoga exercises done with awareness, improvement comes quickly.

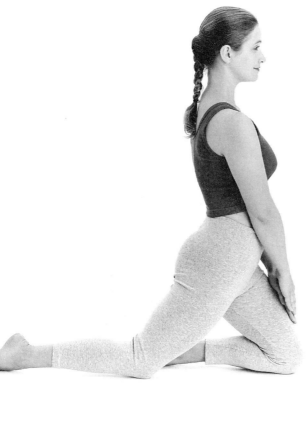

THE DOVE

1 Sit in Vajrasana. Press your hands firmly down on your thighs to keep the spine erect. Lift the sternum (breastbone) and keep it up throughout this sequence. Rise on to your knees as you breathe *in* and stretch your right leg out behind you as far as you can. As you breathe *out*, sit down on your left heel, pushing with your hands to keep the spine upright.

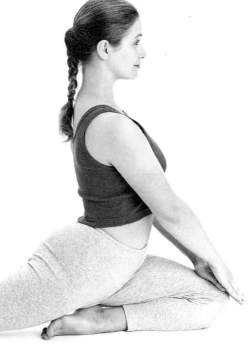

2 Breathe *in* as you raise your right arm to shoulder height in front of you. As you breathe *out* twist the upper body round to the right, bringing the right arm directly above the right foot. Stretch *up* as you breathe *in* and reach *back* as you breathe *out*, improving and holding the pose with each breath. When you have done enough, bring your arm to the front again and lower it. Press both hands on to the thighs to hold the spine upright.

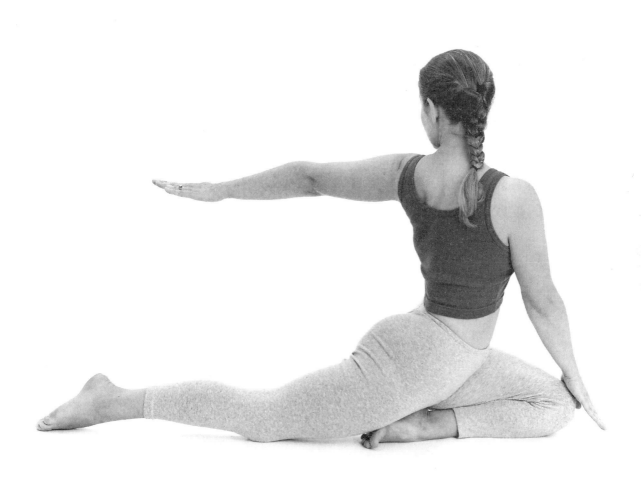

3 Breathing *in*, raise your left arm up in front of you at shoulder height. As you breathe *out*, twist this time to the left as far as you can, taking a few breaths to improve your position. Slowly and gently return to the Vajrasana position and rest there a moment, before repeating the whole sequence sitting on your right foot with the left leg stretched behind you.

Take care to work both sides equally. Finally, rest in whichever position your body feels that it needs.

WATCHPOINT: The most important consideration in the preceding two sequences is to keep the spine upright all the time! This will prepare you for the next sequence.

CRESCENT MOON

1 Bring your hands into the 'Indian greeting' position, palms together, fingers pointing up and thumbs towards your heart. As you breathe *in*, kneel up.

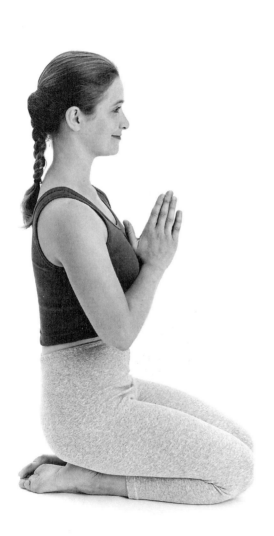

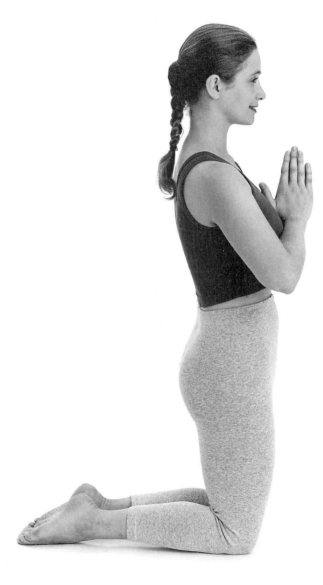

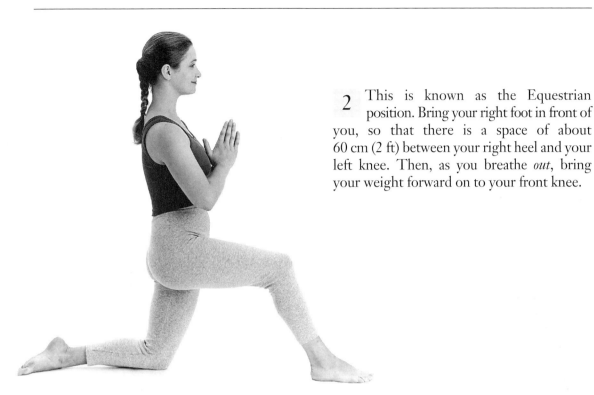

2 This is known as the Equestrian position. Bring your right foot in front of you, so that there is a space of about 60 cm (2 ft) between your right heel and your left knee. Then, as you breathe *out*, bring your weight forward on to your front knee.

WATCHPOINT: If there is not enough space between your front heel and your back knee you will find the front knee coming forward of the front ankle. This is incorrect! If there is too much space, the front knee will come behind the front ankle. This is also incorrect! Much of your body weight is transferred to the ground, in this position, through your front knee and ankle. Therefore it is essential to keep 'joint over joint' for safe use of the body. You will need to make careful adjustment to get the distance right for you; as you become more supple, you will find that the distance needs to be readjusted. The hips should be slung low, as if on carriage springs, with the spine rising up out of them.

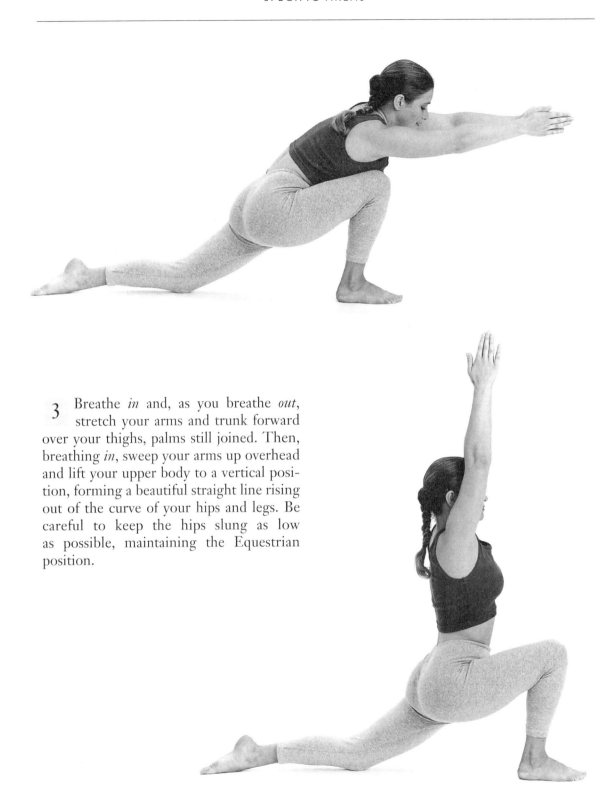

3 Breathe *in* and, as you breathe *out*, stretch your arms and trunk forward over your thighs, palms still joined. Then, breathing *in*, sweep your arms up overhead and lift your upper body to a vertical position, forming a beautiful straight line rising out of the curve of your hips and legs. Be careful to keep the hips slung as low as possible, maintaining the Equestrian position.

4 Breathe *in* and, as you breathe *out*, arch the upper part of the body and the arms backward, forming the line of the Crescent Moon from your fingers, through your body and down to your back foot. Hold and improve your position with deep, slow breathing until you become tired.

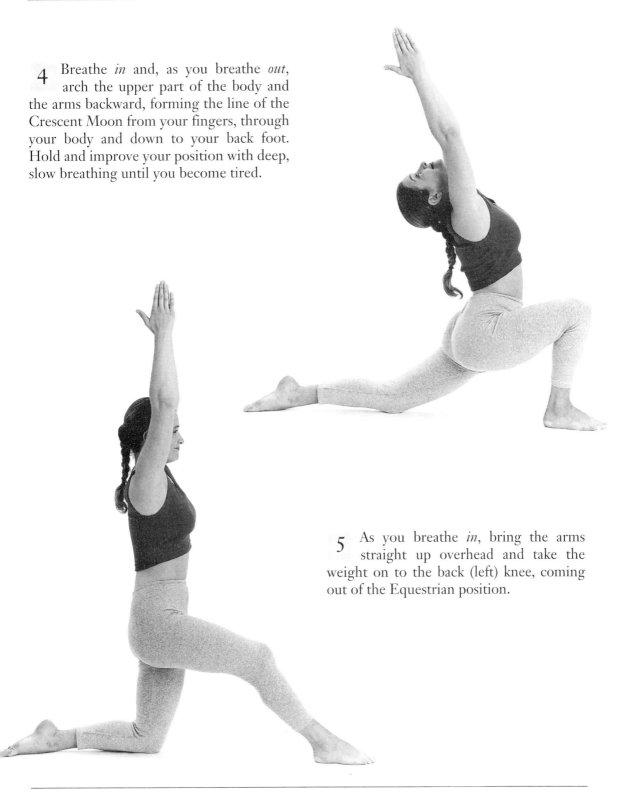

5 As you breathe *in*, bring the arms straight up overhead and take the weight on to the back (left) knee, coming out of the Equestrian position.

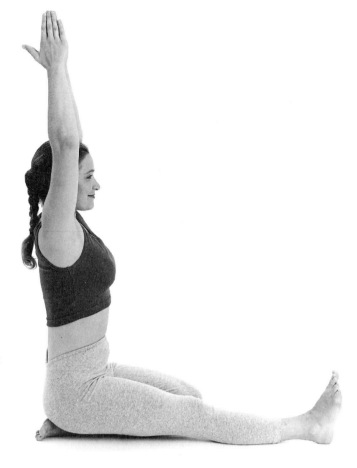

6 As you breathe *out*, sit down on the left foot (turning the toes inwards to make a comfortable 'cushion'). Breathe *in* and stretch *up* through the spine and arms. Flex your front (right) foot and turn the toes *up*.

7 As you breathe *out*, bring your arms and trunk forward, in a straight line, as far as you can. Breathe *in*. As you breathe *out* again, relax down into the Forward Bend position. Breathe slowly and deeply. You may be able to keep your hands together in the 'Indian greeting', hooking them over your flexed foot. If you cannot reach that far, place them one on each side of your outstretched leg, palms *up*.

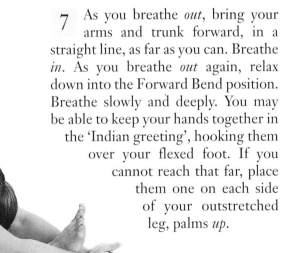

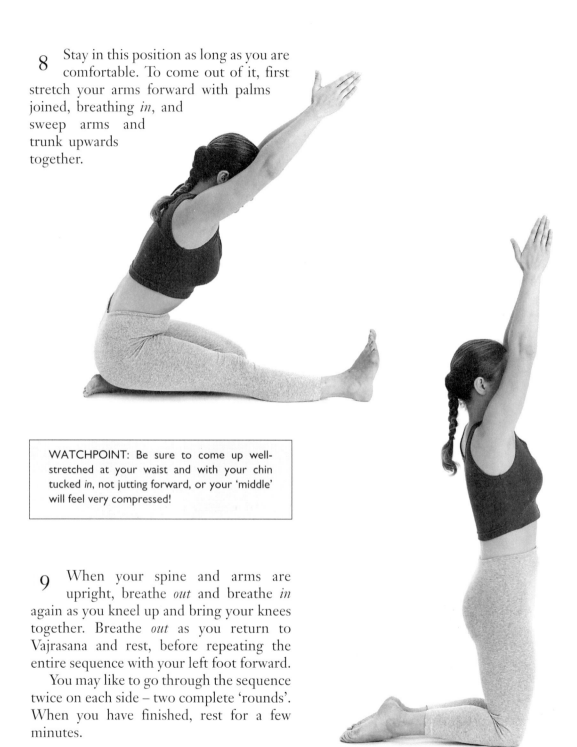

8 Stay in this position as long as you are comfortable. To come out of it, first stretch your arms forward with palms joined, breathing *in*, and sweep arms and trunk upwards together.

WATCHPOINT: Be sure to come up well-stretched at your waist and with your chin tucked *in*, not jutting forward, or your 'middle' will feel very compressed!

9 When your spine and arms are upright, breathe *out* and breathe *in* again as you kneel up and bring your knees together. Breathe *out* as you return to Vajrasana and rest, before repeating the entire sequence with your left foot forward.

You may like to go through the sequence twice on each side – two complete 'rounds'. When you have finished, rest for a few minutes.

EQUESTRIAN TWIST

1 Get your hips properly 'slung' between your front upright knee and your back knee on the floor. Breathing *in*, bring your arms *up* overhead to get a good upright line in the spine.

2 Breathe *out* and bring your arms to the sides at shoulder level, palms down. Breathe *in* again and, as you breathe *out*, twist your trunk to the side, keeping your arms stretched out. Breathe *in* to face front and *out* to twist to the other side.

You may like to repeat the twist to both sides several times more. When you have finished, change legs, bringing the other knee forward, and repeat the sequence on the other side for the same number of times. Then rest in the Child (see page 56).

WATCHPOINT: All movements done from the Equestrian position are strenuous! Proceed only as far and as fast as you feel comfortable. Besides the yoga of body, breath, focus and relaxation, there is also a strong element of balance. Good preparatory movements would be Antelope (see Chapter 4) and JackKnife (see Chapter 6).

CHAPTER 11

TWISTING MOVEMENTS

For a healthy spine

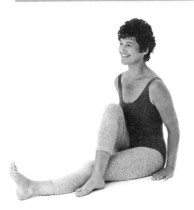

HAVING WORKED HARD to develop a strong foundation, we are now able to express ourselves fully and uniquely as who we are. The sequences that follow bring out the graceful individuality of yoga, yet are easier to do than they look. Twisting movements affect the entire spine. The ones that follow are not as demanding as the strong sequences in Chapters 9 and 10, but rely upon co-ordination, overall strength, suppleness, focus and relaxation. Their effect is subtle, enhancing energy and a feeling of joyful wellbeing throughout your whole self.

The first flowing movements start from Tadasana. You will need to be aware of your body as a whole, standing tall and strong, yet supple.

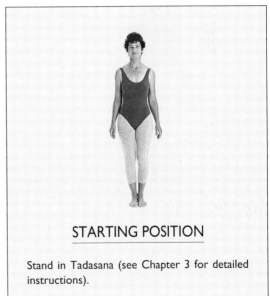

STARTING POSITION

Stand in Tadasana (see Chapter 3 for detailed instructions).

LINE-UP TWIST

1 Place your left toes on the floor a few centimetres (inches) to the right of your right foot. Stand tall with your weight on your right foot. Twist your trunk to the left, bringing both hands up to eye level. Join the thumb and forefinger of each hand, to make two circles. Stretch your left hand as far away from you and round to the left as possible. Turn your head to look to the left. Line up your right hand so that you can gaze through both 'circles' at once into the far distance – or some other world!

2 Lift your left toes from the floor, sweep your left foot around behind your right foot and stand on it firmly, at the same time shifting your weight and raising your right heel from the floor. While you are doing this, simultaneously twist your trunk around to the right. At the same time stretch your right arm out and behind you, lining up the two 'circles' with your right hand farthest away. Turn your head to the right to gaze through both 'circles'.

Once you have sorted out the movements themselves, you can let them flow 'on the breath'. Breathe *in* as you change

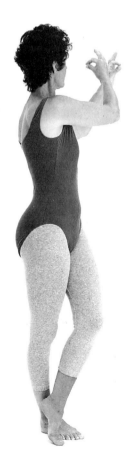

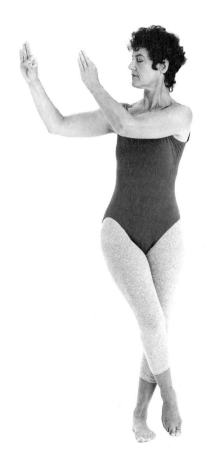

your foot position and stand firm and tall. Breathe *out* as you twist the trunk, neck and head and align your arms to gaze through the 'circles' made by your forefinger and thumb on each hand. As you repeat these graceful movements, feel that they are a part of your breath, a physical expression of the music within you. Needless to say, you need to be both focused and relaxed in your mind, in order to 'flow'.

After a few twists, repeat all the movements to the other side, by moving your right foot around your left leg, rather than your left foot around your right leg. Notice the difference in your balance and fluidity.

When you have finished, stand in Tadasana with your eyes closed, feeling the swirling of energy inside you. You have been doing a 'moving meditation'.

RISHI'S TWIST

A rishi was someone who retired to the forests of Ancient India to meditate. Presumably he also needed some exercise! This sequence should, like the last one, be done 'from the inside out'.

1 Stand tall in Tadasana. Place your legs about 90 cm (3 ft) apart, with the feet and knees turned out at a comfortable angle. Your legs will remain straight throughout. Join your palms near the heart in the 'Indian greeting' position.

2 Slide your left hand down the inside of your right leg, bending forward and twisting from the waist upwards as far round to the right as you can. At the same time, bring your right arm up, fingers pointing to

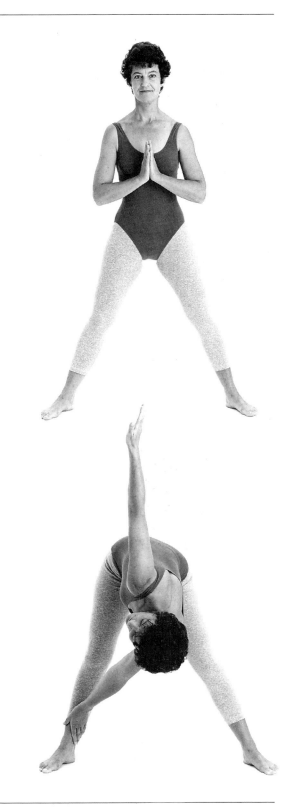

the ceiling immediately above your head and palm facing to the right. Open your right shoulder as much as possible.

To come up, bring your top hand down and your bottom hand up to meet at the heart in the 'Indian greeting' position as you untwist your spine and lift the trunk, still centred between your open legs. Repeat, twisting to the left.

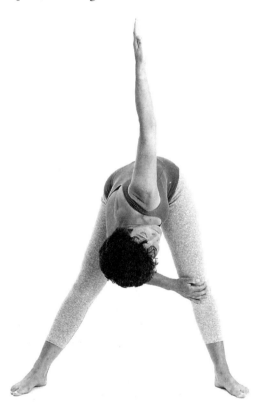

Once you can get smoothly in and out of this posture, 'flow' with the breath. Bring your head down and arm up as you breathe *out*. Come up centring yourself at the heart, as you breathe *in*. Repeat several times on each side, concentrating on the position of every part of your body and enjoying the smooth co-ordination of your breath and

movements. When you have finished, stand with eyes closed in Tadasana, feeling both exhilarated and centred.

WATCHPOINT: Keep in line! You may need a friend to check. Your head should be down, centred between your legs, with your shoulder immediately above it and the arm stretching up vertically. It is very easy to forget to open the shoulder, and just wave the hand overhead and hope for the best!

Now for some gentle twists that make you feel very 'inward'.

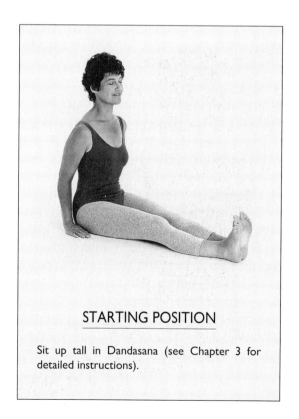

STARTING POSITION

Sit up tall in Dandasana (see Chapter 3 for detailed instructions).

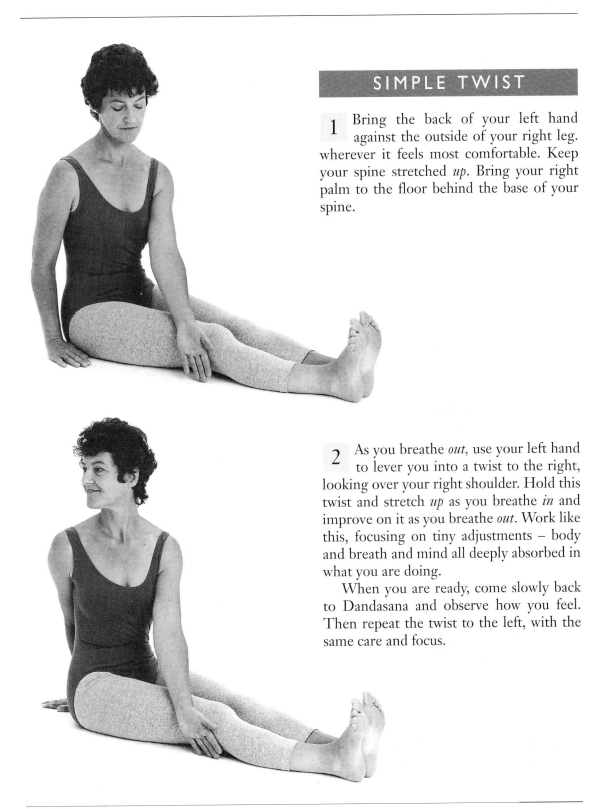

SIMPLE TWIST

1 Bring the back of your left hand against the outside of your right leg. wherever it feels most comfortable. Keep your spine stretched *up*. Bring your right palm to the floor behind the base of your spine.

2 As you breathe *out*, use your left hand to lever you into a twist to the right, looking over your right shoulder. Hold this twist and stretch *up* as you breathe *in* and improve on it as you breathe *out*. Work like this, focusing on tiny adjustments – body and breath and mind all deeply absorbed in what you are doing.

When you are ready, come slowly back to Dandasana and observe how you feel. Then repeat the twist to the left, with the same care and focus.

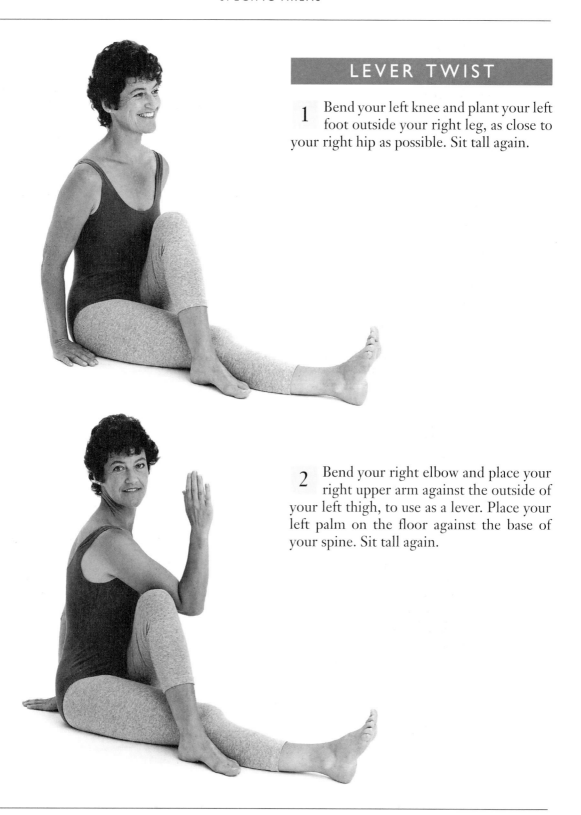

LEVER TWIST

1 Bend your left knee and plant your left foot outside your right leg, as close to your right hip as possible. Sit tall again.

2 Bend your right elbow and place your right upper arm against the outside of your left thigh, to use as a lever. Place your left palm on the floor against the base of your spine. Sit tall again.

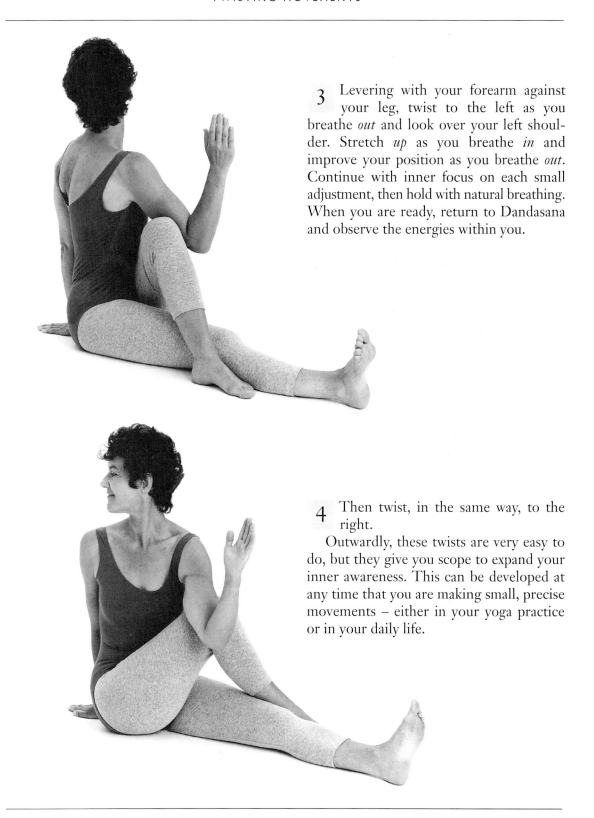

3 Levering with your forearm against your leg, twist to the left as you breathe *out* and look over your left shoulder. Stretch *up* as you breathe *in* and improve your position as you breathe *out*. Continue with inner focus on each small adjustment, then hold with natural breathing. When you are ready, return to Dandasana and observe the energies within you.

4 Then twist, in the same way, to the right.

Outwardly, these twists are very easy to do, but they give you scope to expand your inner awareness. This can be developed at any time that you are making small, precise movements – either in your yoga practice or in your daily life.

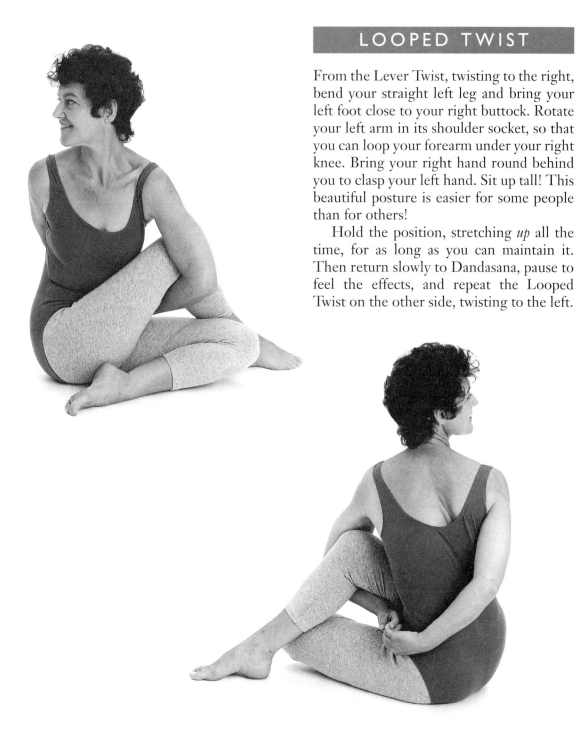

LOOPED TWIST

From the Lever Twist, twisting to the right, bend your straight left leg and bring your left foot close to your right buttock. Rotate your left arm in its shoulder socket, so that you can loop your forearm under your right knee. Bring your right hand round behind you to clasp your left hand. Sit up tall! This beautiful posture is easier for some people than for others!

Hold the position, stretching *up* all the time, for as long as you can maintain it. Then return slowly to Dandasana, pause to feel the effects, and repeat the Looped Twist on the other side, twisting to the left.

CHAPTER 12

OPENING UP

Arching and inverting the body

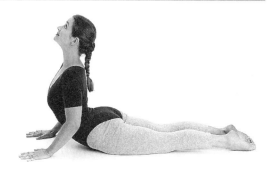

LIFE IS A CHALLENGE which can be met in two ways. One way is to reject those parts of it with which we do not feel comfortable, and to pretend that we are not hurt or angry or isolated – or whatever it is that we actually feel! The other, the way of yoga, is to accept things as they are, including our own feelings.

As you work through the exercises in this book, you are frequently reminded to stop and observe quietly how you feel at the end of a sequence. In this way you get to know yourself from the inside, rather than relying upon the distorted impressions that you receive from other people. Many of us simply do not know how we feel about anything, only how we have been told we should feel! When we fail to react as prescribed by others, we get confused and lose confidence in ourselves. Insight comes with regular yoga practice, particularly the 'yoga of observation'. Gradually we become

more our own person and less reliant on others to tell us who we are.

Opening the chest seems to open us up to our own feelings as well. Every time you stretch up through the spine and lift your sternum (breastbone) you become more 'real' to yourself – and therefore everyone else becomes more real as well!

Arching the spine opens the heart.

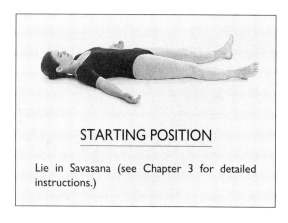

STARTING POSITION

Lie in Savasana (see Chapter 3 for detailed instructions.)

PRONE POSE

Roll over on to your front, with your forehead to the floor, legs straight and feet together. Bend your elbows, keeping them tucked in at shoulder width ('joint over joint'). Place your palms at heart level, either side of your chest.

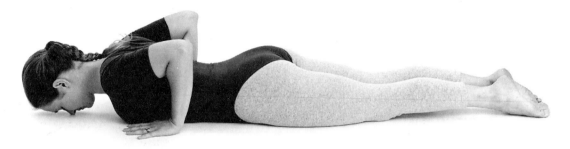

ARM LIFT

From the Prone Pose above, raise your arms behind you and clasp your hands firmly together. 'Pull' your upper trunk up and back by stretching your hands up and towards your feet. Hopefully your chest will rise from the floor! Feel the muscles working in your upper back, and the weight of your lower abdomen and pelvis supporting you against the floor. Keep your legs straight and feet together on the floor.

When you get tired, return to the Prone Pose and repeat after a short rest. If you find this exercise difficult, do please practise it regularly! It will soon get easier. You will need strength in your upper back for the inverted poses (see pages 114–16).

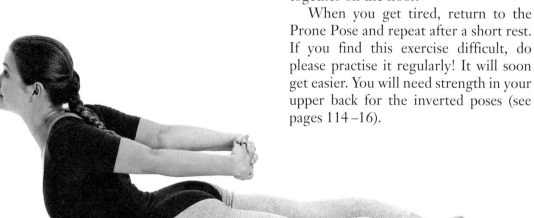

MODIFIED COBRA

1 From the Prone Pose opposite, take your hands forward, elbows still in line with your shoulders for safe lifting. Place your elbows directly under your shoulders, with forearms on the floor in front of you. This will raise your chest from the floor.

> WATCHPOINT: In all versions of the Cobra it is important to keep your neck long and the shoulders *down*. It is very easy – and quite pointless! – to hunch your shoulders and push into your hands to lift your upper body, bypassing the upper back muscles altogether!

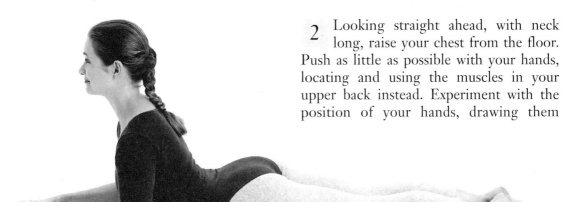

2 Looking straight ahead, with neck long, raise your chest from the floor. Push as little as possible with your hands, locating and using the muscles in your upper back instead. Experiment with the position of your hands, drawing them

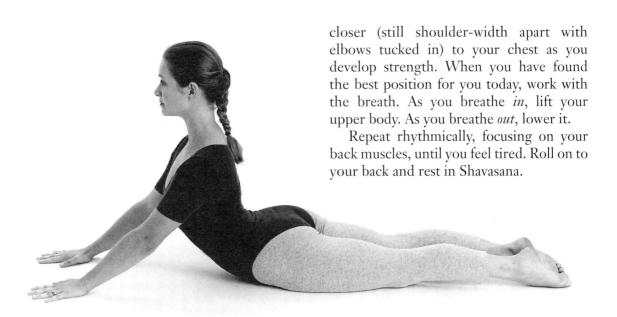

closer (still shoulder-width apart with elbows tucked in) to your chest as you develop strength. When you have found the best position for you today, work with the breath. As you breathe *in*, lift your upper body. As you breathe *out*, lower it.

Repeat rhythmically, focusing on your back muscles, until you feel tired. Roll on to your back and rest in Shavasana.

CLASSICAL COBRA

1 From the Prone Pose above, lift your upper body as you breathe *in*. Hold the position as you breathe *out*. Lift a fraction more as you breathe *in* and hold as you breathe *out*. Focus on the muscles in your upper back and avoid putting all your weight on to your hands. Continue working like this, synchronized with your breathing.

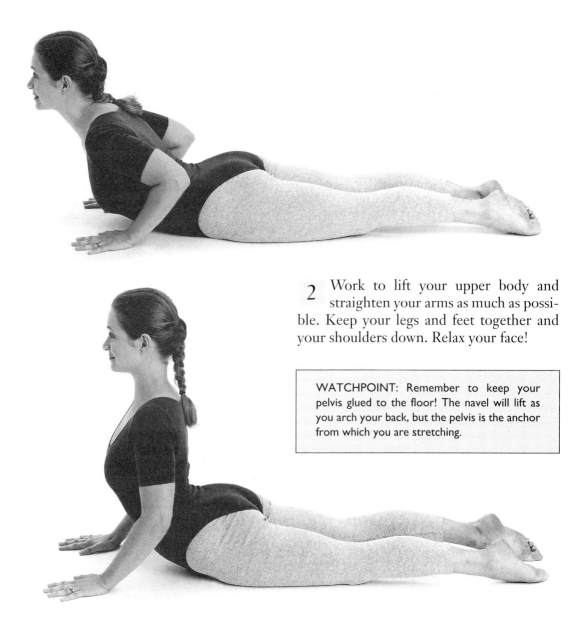

2 Work to lift your upper body and straighten your arms as much as possible. Keep your legs and feet together and your shoulders down. Relax your face!

WATCHPOINT: Remember to keep your pelvis glued to the floor! The navel will lift as you arch your back, but the pelvis is the anchor from which you are stretching.

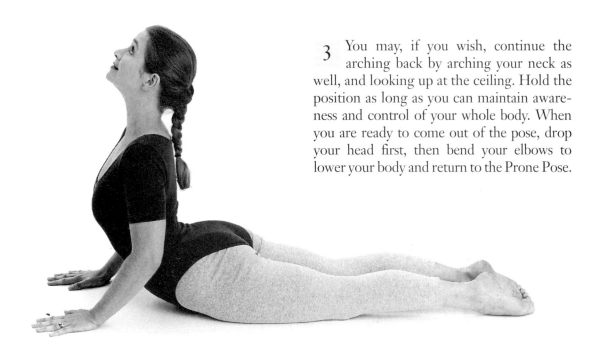

3 You may, if you wish, continue the arching back by arching your neck as well, and looking up at the ceiling. Hold the position as long as you can maintain awareness and control of your whole body. When you are ready to come out of the pose, drop your head first, then bend your elbows to lower your body and return to the Prone Pose.

KNEELING STRETCH

From the Prone Pose you may like to go into the Kneeling Stretch to rest.

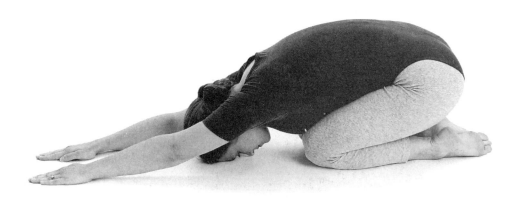

DRAGONFLY

This is a lovely balancing pose, as well as a back arch.

1   Start in the Prone Pose. Bring your chin to the floor, stretching the front of your neck. Raise your left leg into the air, keeping it straight. Bend your right knee and rest your straight left knee on the sole of your right foot. Raise your arms up straight behind you, like wings, stretching into your fingertips.

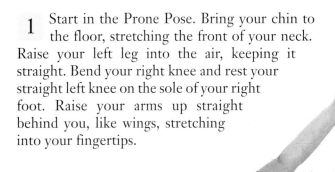

2   As you breathe *in*, lift your head and (if possible) your upper chest – and 'fly'! Breathe naturally and hold the position as long as you can. Return to the Prone Pose. Repeat with right leg raised. Then rest in the Kneeling Stretch, before returning to Shavasana.

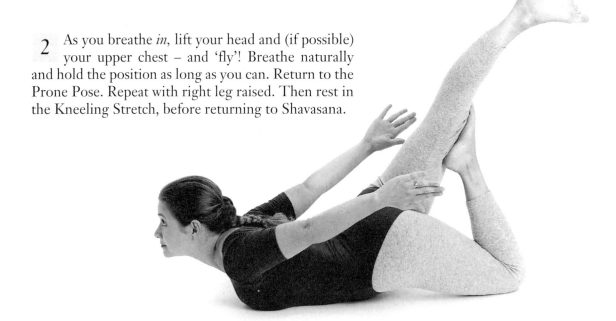

PELVIC TILT

1 Bend your knees and plant your feet as close to your buttocks as possible, a hip's-width apart ('joint over joint') for safe lifting. Turn your toes in slightly to lift your arches and take the weight on to the outsides of your feet. Bring your arms close to your body with palms down, to help to support your weight as you lift.

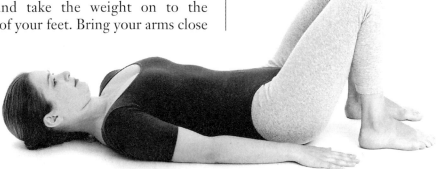

2 Keep your chin tucked in, neck long, and waist glued to the floor. Breathe *in*. As you breathe *out*, lift your coccyx (tailbone) from the floor, tilting your pelvis. This is a very slight movement, but it does wonders for your pelvic floor muscles and your overall posture. Breathe in as you lower your coccyx and breathe *out* as you raise it again. This time, try to 'suck up and in', contracting the pelvic floor muscles up into the lower abdomen. Relax as you breathe *in* and bring the coccyx back to the floor.

Repeat this several times, focusing on your pelvic floor all the time. Then hold the lifted position and the pelvic floor contraction, with natural breathing, for as long as you can. Lower and rest.

If your pelvic floor muscles are weak – often from stretching in childbirth – gynaecological and urinary problems can result, because the organs are not being held in their proper position. It is a valuable insurance for future health and comfort to work on this area now.

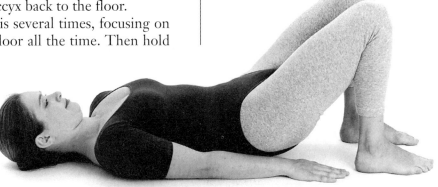

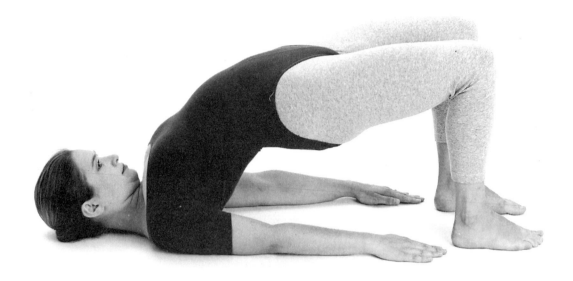

BRIDGE-PEELING

Start in the Pelvic Tilt position above. Make sure that your arms are alongside your body, with palms down, and that your feet are strongly 'planted' a hip's-width apart, as close to your buttocks as possible. Turn your toes in again slightly, if they have moved, so that you are ready to lift your spine off the floor. Breathe *in*. As you breathe *out*, lift your coccyx (tailbone) off the floor into the Pelvic Tilt and contract your pelvic floor muscles. Hold this contraction.

As you breathe *in*, lift your spine slowly off the floor, vertebra by vertebra. Keep your mind focused on your spine as it moves. Get in touch with the feel of each vertebra. When you need to breathe *out*, pause in your lifting and tighten your pelvic floor muscles again. Continue 'peeling'

your vertebrae off the floor as you breathe *in* again.

WATCHPOINT: You are about to bring your heart higher than your head, in a partially inverted position. Were you comfortable in the other upside-down positions you have tried so far? These were Dog (see Chapter 7), Woodchopper (see Chapter 8), Extended Standing Forward Bend (see Chapter 9) and Rishi's Twist (see Chapter 10). Were you happy upside down in all these positions? If not, go very cautiously from now on in Bridge-peeling and do not attempt any of the postures that follow in this chapter.

If you are comfortable, continue working like this until your entire spine, up to the shoulders, is raised high off the floor. Use your upper back muscles to push your sternum (breastbone) up against your chin, which should still be tucked in.

Hold this position, breathing naturally, until you feel tired. Then lower your spine to the floor very slowly, with natural breathing, focusing on each vertebra as it contacts the floor.

Some parts of your spine may feel much more alive and responsive than other parts. This is natural. Focusing on the spine will gradually bring much more 'out into the open' that which we were previously hiding from ourselves. Strength and awareness in the spine is far more than physical!

HIGH BRIDGE

You may like to stretch one leg up towards the ceiling to help you to get a feeling of lightness as well as of uplift. If so, slide your foot along the floor, lift that leg and straighten it as you stretch it up. Lower in the same way and repeat with the other leg.

WATCHPOINT: Do not let the hips tilt or drop down as you stretch your leg up.

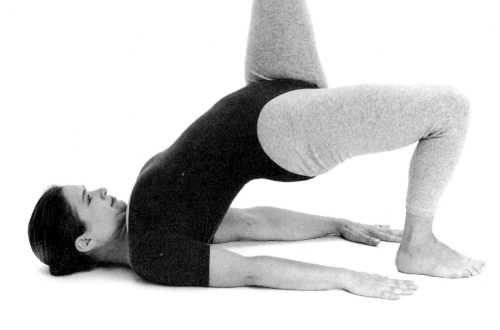

INVERTED POSE

The yoga inverted poses are very famous, and beginners often want to try them. However, they do require a great deal of preparation with the kind of postures described throughout this book.

They also require developed internal awareness on the part of the practitioner. Is it safe for you to invert your body? By now, you should know. You should also immediately recognize any warning signals, and be prepared to come out – at once – of whatever position you are in.

Up to now, you have been introduced to some partially inverted positions which are elements of a longer sequence. You have moved easily in and out of them on the breath. You have not held them unless you were perfectly comfortable in them. You have certainly not been 'trapped' in any of them!

This is not the case with true inverted poses. They are designed to be 'fixed', so that you can stay in them for several minutes at least. So, before you embark upon them, please be *absolutely sure* that you are comfortable upside down!

Inverted poses are usually done at the end of the exercise session, before breathing exercises and deep relaxation, or a short meditation.

1 To get into the Inverted Pose, start in the Pelvic Tilt position. Now lift your feet off the floor, bringing your knees towards your chest. Breathe *in*, and roll your hips up over your head as you breathe *out*, placing your hands on your spine and moving them upwards to support you as you roll up. Breathing naturally, work your hips upwards to be directly over your shoulders ('joint over joint'), pushing with your palms against your spine, fingers pointing up. Straighten your spine into a straight line, using the muscles of your upper back.

If you cannot get your back straight, come down again as you went up, supported by your hands on your spine and your upper arms on the floor. You will need to do a lot more Bridge-peeling (see page

WATCHPOINT: Keep your elbows close to your body to take your weight while you are inverted. They should stay in line with your shoulders and not be allowed to splay outwards.

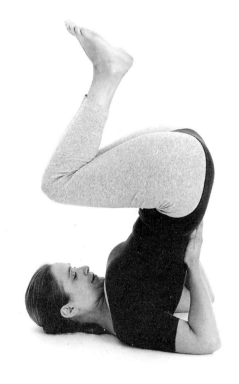

112) to strengthen your upper back before you embark upon inverted postures.

2 When you have worked your back into a straight line over your shoulders, slowly bring both your knees on to your forehead and rest them there. Breathe slowly and deeply. Count your breaths. Allow 16 slow breaths – the time it takes for your heart to get used to being upside down! – before making any further movement (except rolling down if you feel tired or uncomfortable).

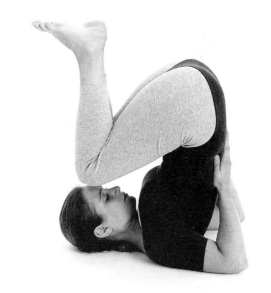

INVERTED DRAGONFLY

After your 16 breaths in the Inverted Pose, gingerly raise one leg up straight, keeping your balance, and place your knee upon the sole of the foot of your bent leg. Remain in this position, counting your breaths, then bend your straight leg and bring your knee back to rest on your forehead. Repeat for the same number of breaths with the other leg straight, then return to the Inverted Pose and come back from there to the Pelvic Tilt position (see page 111).

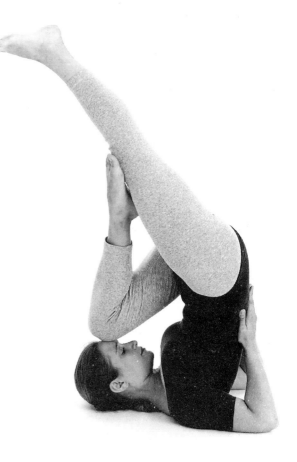

POSE OF TRANQUILLITY

This is a wonderful pose, with many of the benefits of the classical inverted poses without being nearly so demanding to hold. Start from the Inverted Dragonfly above. Very gingerly, keeping your balance, remove from your back the arm that is on the same side as the straight leg. Transfer the weight of your straight leg from your opposite knee into the palm of your free hand. Straighten that arm. Pause to regain your balance.

Then take your other hand from your back and bring it into position to accept the bent knee, as you straighten it. Straighten both arms and both legs. You are now balancing on the T-shape of your shoulders and neck. You may need a friend to hold your toes and give you confidence! Remain in this position for as long as possible, breathing naturally and resting deeply.

When you are ready to come out of the pose, do so very slowly and gently. Return to the Inverted Pose, then to the Pelvic Tilt position. Rest there for a while and let your heart settle the right way up.

You may feel like arching your back and easing your neck with the Back Arching Release (see Chapter 6), before lying in Shavasana.

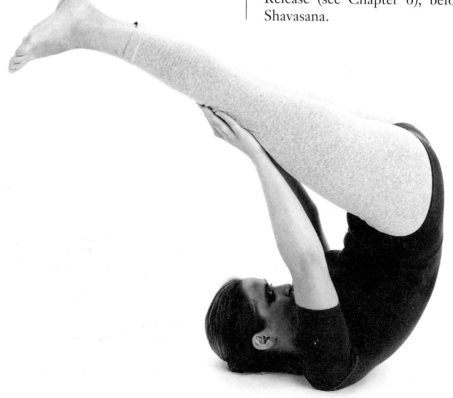

CHAPTER 13

KEEPING THE MIND IN THE BODY

Breathing, meditation and relaxation

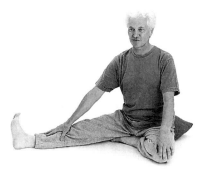

BREATHING EXERCISES usually come after the physical exercises, although breath awareness is always an integral part of yoga. Some breathing exercises, however, fit comfortably into a rest period, either at the beginning – to settle one after a hectic day, perhaps – or somewhere in the middle of a session when one needs a pause after strong physical exertion.

Lying in Shavasana, watch the natural flow of the breath for a while. Then deepen the breath a little, keeping it relaxed. If focusing on your breathing makes you

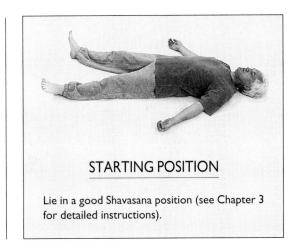

STARTING POSITION

Lie in a good Shavasana position (see Chapter 3 for detailed instructions).

nervous, stop. Take your mind instead to some part of your body connected with breathing, such as your nostrils. Here you can feel the air passing in and out.

When you have relaxed once more, take your attention back to your breathing and deepen it a little. Alternate between attention on your nostrils and attention on your breathing, until your breath stops being 'shy' at being observed. Five minutes – regularly – is long enough to start with. Just keep relaxed!

This is a good practice at the start of a yoga session. The next stage is to lengthen the breath *out* a little more than the breath *in*. You can count slowly as you breathe *in* and add a bit as you breathe *out* – always without any strain. Changing breathing habits is a slow process.

Once you are used to increasing the length of your breath *out* at will, you will find that you do this automatically in your posture work. You often stretch *up* through the spine as you breathe *in*, and then move on a much slower breath *out*. This becomes the natural way to synchronize breath and movement.

HARA BREATHING

1 From Shavasana, bend your knees and bring the soles of your feet together, as close to your buttocks as possible. Let your knees flop to the side. Bring your arms up overhead and clasp your hands loosely together, several centimetres (inches) above your head. This position 'opens' the front of the body, both in the abdomen and the chest. Breathe slowly and deeply, feeling the movement of energy in the Hara (below the navel). This is a revitalizing type of breathing.

WATCHPOINT: Keep your waist down against the floor and your chin tucked in, so that your spine is long and relaxed. Your elbows should rest on the floor.

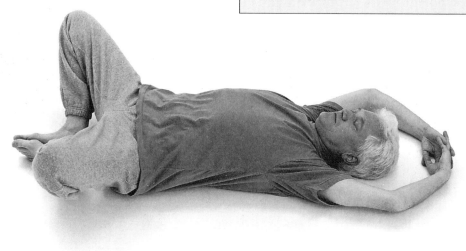

2 If your pectoral (chest) muscles are very tight, your elbows may lift from the floor when you clasp your hands. If so, unclasp them and relax them either side of your head. The 'Universal Pose' (see Chapter 5) works wonders on tight shoulder and chest muscles!

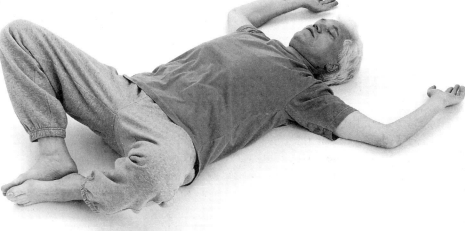

HEART BREATHING

After practising Hara Breathing for a few minutes, change the position of your knees and feet. Bring the knees together (gently!) and plant the feet as wide apart as possible, close to the buttocks. This position 'closes' the abdominal area, so that energy is concentrated in the heart area only. Breathe deeply – you will feel a wonderful peaceful-ness pervading you. After a while, return to Shavasana for a moment, before continuing your yoga session.

As with Hara Breathing, change your arm position if you feel overstretched with your hands clasped. Release and separate them. These two breathing exercises can come as a natural break between dynamic sequences.

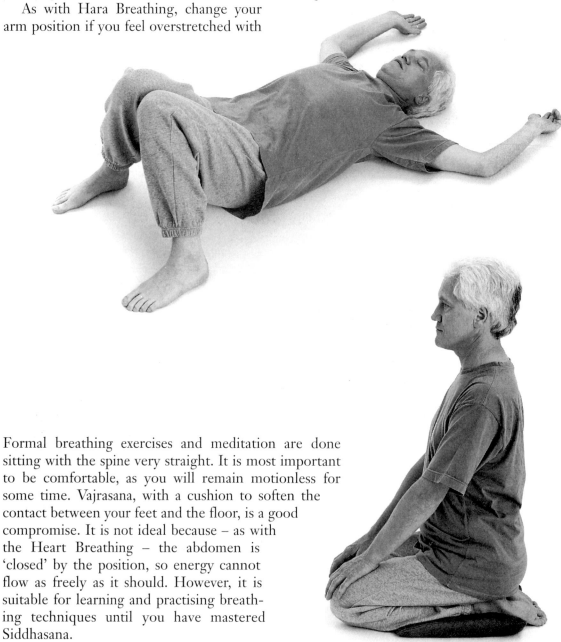

Formal breathing exercises and meditation are done sitting with the spine very straight. It is most important to be comfortable, as you will remain motionless for some time. Vajrasana, with a cushion to soften the contact between your feet and the floor, is a good compromise. It is not ideal because – as with the Heart Breathing – the abdomen is 'closed' by the position, so energy cannot flow as freely as it should. However, it is suitable for learning and practising breath-ing techniques until you have mastered Siddhasana.

SIDDHASANA

This is one of the classical postures for breathing exercises and meditation. It is well worth persevering to learn it, as it is extremely comfortable and secure once it is mastered. The abdomen and chest are both 'open' in this pose, so energy can flow freely. You will probably need a cushion.

The halfway stages are quite easy.

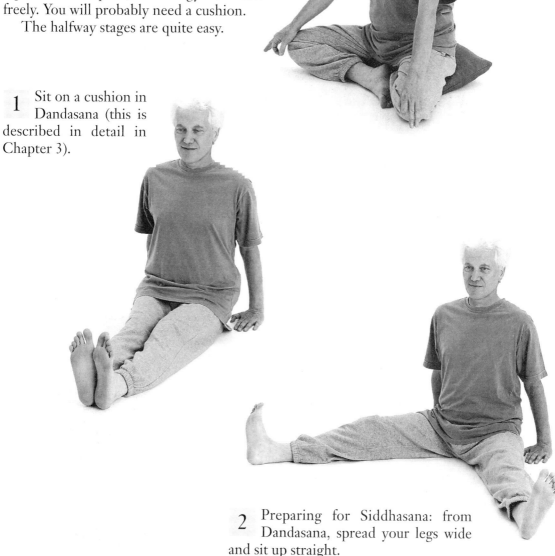

1 Sit on a cushion in Dandasana (this is described in detail in Chapter 3).

2 Preparing for Siddhasana: from Dandasana, spread your legs wide and sit up straight.

3 Still sitting up very straight, bend your left knee and bring the sole of your left foot against the top of your right thigh, with the heel pressing into the base of your pelvis.

WATCHPOINT: Your bent knee should always be in contact with the floor. If it is not, sit on more cushions and/or firm foam blocks, until it is.

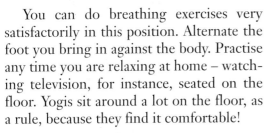

You can do breathing exercises very satisfactorily in this position. Alternate the foot you bring in against the body. Practise any time you are relaxing at home – watching television, for instance, seated on the floor. Yogis sit around a lot on the floor, as a rule, because they find it comfortable!

WATCHPOINT: Before you settle yourself for breathing, meditation or relaxation, put on extra clothes or have a blanket to hand. Your body temperature will drop, and you do not want to disturb your concentration by feeling chilled. Get ready now!

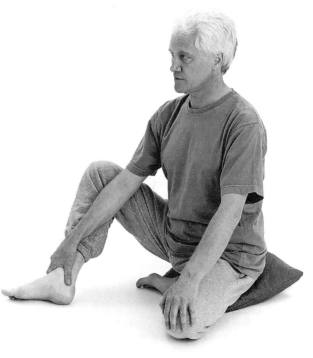

4 To get into the full Siddhasana position, bend your straight leg and bring the foot in towards your body. Place it in front of and touching your other foot, so that both heels are centred and in line and both knees are on the floor. Shuffle forward a little, so that you are almost sitting on the back heel. Alternate the foot you place in

front. You will probably find that one side is easier than the other.

Before long, you may not need the cushion but use it anyway when you plan to remain in Siddhasana for some time.

WATCHPOINT: Siddhasana, once mastered, provides such a firm base that it can be comfortably held for a long time – half an hour or more, with practice. The body literally holds itself up in Siddhasana, provided the knees rest on the floor. Sit on as many cushions and/or firm foam blocks as you need to bring your weight forward on to your knees, so that they are in contact with the floor.

HAND POSITION FOR SIDDHASANA

This pose is 'self-contained', so that energy is built up in the body and cannot escape. Therefore the position of the hands is very important.

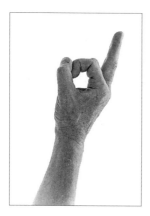

Place the fingernail of the forefinger behind the top joint of the thumb to form

an energy circle. Keep the other three fingers straight and together. Place the left hand, in this position, palm down on your left knee or thigh. Your right hand may be occupied in Alternate Nostril Breathing (see below). If it is not, place it on your right knee or thigh in the same position as the left.

ALTERNATE NOSTRIL BREATHING

This is both a cleansing and balancing breathing exercise. It is a good prelude to deep relaxation in Shavasana, or to seated meditation. You will use your right hand to control the flow of air through your nostrils.

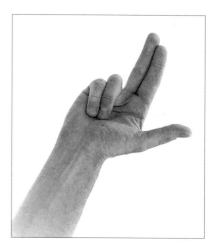

Raise your right hand, with first and second fingers together and straight, and third and fourth fingers curled together into your palm. Place the straight fingers on your forehead, with the thumb beside your right nostril and the third finger beside your left nostril.

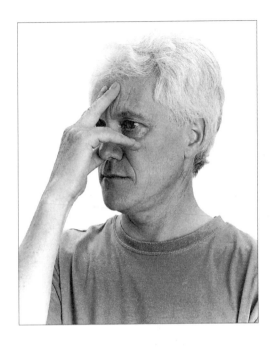

BREATHE AS FOLLOWS:

Breathe *in.*

Close your right nostril with your thumb and breathe *out* through your left nostril only.

Breathe *in* again through your left nostril only.

Close your left nostril with your third finger and open your right nostril.

Breathe *out* through your right nostril only.

Breathe *in* through your right nostril only.

That is one round.

It takes a little time to get fingers and breathing co-ordinated. Take it gently! Get used to sitting and breathing after posture work. Breathe naturally for a few minutes, then practise a few rounds of Alternate Nostril Breathing – just 2 or 3 minutes to start with. You will very quickly feel calm and centred.

> WATCHPOINT: If your mind begins to wander, you may begin to droop, so that your forehead leans on your straight fingers. Push yourself upright again with your fingers. This will restore your concentration!

After you have finished your breathing practice, you can either sit for meditation or lie down for relaxation. The only difference is whether your spine is vertical (meditation) or horizontal (relaxation)! What you do is exactly the same: you will be 'keeping your mind in your body' while your body is motionless, your breathing is natural and your mind is both alert and relaxed.

Sit in Siddhasana (or Vajrasana) on a cushion, for meditation. Close your eyes.

SHAVASANA FOR DEEP RELAXATION

1 Put your extra clothes on before you lie down. (See Chapter 3 for more detailed instructions on Shavasana). Remember that you will be lying completely motionless on the floor for 10–15 minutes. If you find that this is uncomfortable, you can place a cushion strategically. (See opposite.)

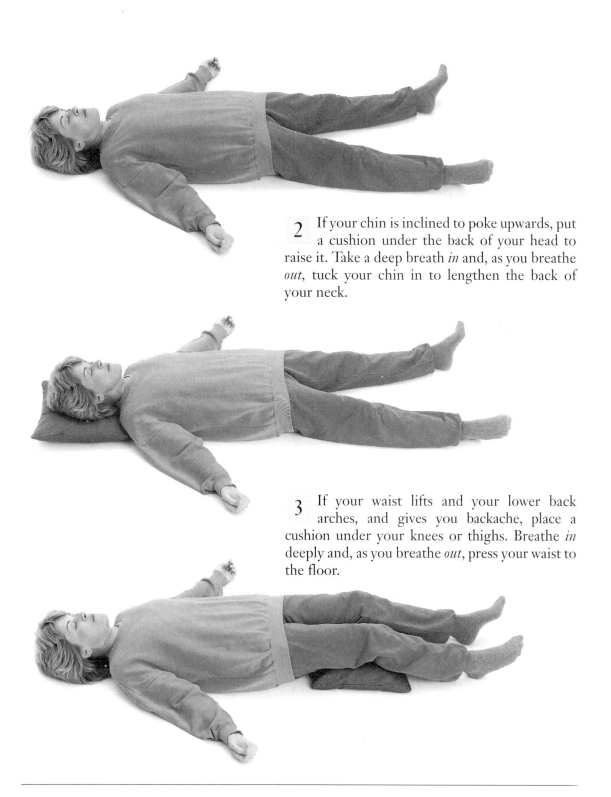

2 If your chin is inclined to poke upwards, put a cushion under the back of your head to raise it. Take a deep breath *in* and, as you breathe *out*, tuck your chin in to lengthen the back of your neck.

3 If your waist lifts and your lower back arches, and gives you backache, place a cushion under your knees or thighs. Breathe *in* deeply and, as you breathe *out*, press your waist to the floor.

MEDITATION/DEEP RELAXATION

SIT OR LIE COMFORTABLY

CLOSE YOUR EYES

STEP 1
Close your eyes and keep your eyeballs as still as possible.
Stillness in the body, especially the eyes, brings stillness to the mind.

STEP 2
Move your attention from your eyeballs to your body.
Connect with many different parts of your body in turn.
Observe the stillness of your body.

STEP 3
Move your attention to your breathing.
Breathe naturally, keeping your mind focused on the breathing process.
Observe the feeling as the air comes into your nostrils from outside your body.
Watch the passage of air into your lungs and out again.

STEP 4
Find your still centre in your heart space.
See a small flame burning there.
It burns steadily, without movement.
Watch this flame for a while.

STEP 5
Feel peacefulness within and around you.
Be grateful that you have found peace within your own self.
Recognize it.
Know that it is always there for you, whenever you need it.

BACK TO STEP 4
Watch the flame again for a while.

BACK TO STEP 3
Watch your breathing again for a while.

BACK TO STEP 2
Become aware again of your body.
When you are ready, move your fingers and toes.
Rotate your wrists and ankles and your neck.
Stretch slowly and gently.

BACK TO STEP 1
Open your eyes.
Look around you.
Sit up slowly (if you are lying down).

'CLOSING' RITUAL
Bring your hands into the 'Indian greeting' position, thumbs to your heart.
Bring your hands to the floor to 'ground' you, in the Kneeling Stretch.
Be sure you are wide awake before you get up.

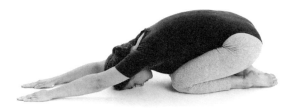

You will see, from the above, that there is no 'thinking' – only observing, feeling and visualizing. This gives the mind a wonderful rest! If thoughts interrupt you, do not fight them. Just look at them calmly until they go away, embarrassed!

Sometimes sudden insights come. Write them down before you forget them, as they can bring profound changes in your attitudes and perceptions.

Work with the above 'steps' a little at a time, always coming out in reverse order.

Soon they will become so familiar that you will follow them automatically as soon as you are comfortably settled.

WATCHPOINT: Do be careful to wait several minutes after you open your eyes before leaving your yoga place. You should never rush out and get on with something else at once – you will feel horribly jangled! It is positively *dangerous* to leap into a car and drive it when you are half awake!

Enjoy your yoga!

INDEX